Nursing in Conflict

Other titles by the authors

Community Care and Severe Physical Disability
Patricia Owens

Paying for Welfare, The Future of the Welfare State
Howard Glennerster

Planning for Priority Groups
Howard Glennerster

Nursing in Conflict

———————— ◆ ————————

Patricia Owens
formerly Research Officer
London School of Economics

and

Howard Glennerster
Professor of Social Administration
London School of Economics

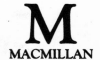

MACMILLAN

First published 1990

Published by
MACMILLAN EDUCATION LTD
Houndmills, Basingstoke, Hampshire RG21 2XS
and London
Companies and representatives
throughout the world

Cover pictures copyright Times Newspapers Ltd
and The Mansell Collection

Typeset by Footnote Graphics,
Warminster, Wilts

Printed in Great Britain by
Billing & Sons
Worcester

British Library Cataloguing in Publication Data
Owens, Patricia
Nursing in conflict.
1. Great Britain. Nursing services. Management
I. Title   II. Glennerster, Howard
610.73'068
ISBN 0–333–51202–2

Contents

———————◆———————

List of tables

———————— ◆ ————————

List of figures

───────── ◆ ─────────

List of abbreviations

◆

A & E	Accident and Emergency Department
CNM	Clinical Nurse Manager
CNO	Chief Nursing Officer
CSM	Clinical Service Manager
DGM	District General Manager
DHA	District Health Authority
DMB	District Management Board
DMS	Director of Midwifery Services
DNA	District Nurse Adviser
DNAC	District Nursing Advisory Committee
DNE	Director of Nurse Education
DNS	Director of Nursing Services
D of H	Department of Health
DQA	Director of Quality Assurance
ENB	English National Board for Nursing, Midwifery and Health Visiting
ITU or CCU	Intensive Care Units or Critical Care Units
NWT RHA	North West Thames Regional Health Authority
RGM	Regional General Manager
RNAC	Regional Nursing Advisory Committee
RND	Regional Nursing Director
SM	Service Manager
SNM	Senior Nurse Manager
UGM	Unit General Manager

Acknowledgements

———— ◆ ————

This research was funded by North West Thames Regional Health Authority to explore nurse management functions after the Griffiths proposals. The initiators of the research were Mrs Pamela Hudson-Bendersky, Regional Nursing Director for NWT, and Professor Howard Glennerster, supported by the Regional General Manager, Mr David Kenny. Throughout the research period, they and members of the Steering Committee have continued to support and advise on the research.

It would be impossible to name all the individuals in NWT region at district level who have helped to make this research project possible, but we are deeply indebted to them all. Sheila Roy, Judith Sear, Frank Powell, Margaret Dorman, Bob Nessling, Brian Hambleton, June Swan, Ann Mace, David Pennell, Pat Fletcher, Joy Byatt, Diana Juniper, Meiriona William, Katherine Conway-Nicholls, Judith Bryant, Anita Cox, Moira Stansfield, Jean Bailey and Aidine Phillips smoothed the way for the researchers, as did the General Managers in all districts. At LSE we wish to thank Sheila Gatiss who assisted in collecting material for the research in two districts, and Angela Kimberley, Carol Whitwill and Julie Grove-Hills who worked very hard to put the results into print.

Introduction

————————— ◆ —————————

Time present and time past
Are both perhaps present in time future,
And time future contained in time past.
(T. S. Eliot)

This book is about NHS management and its relationship with the nursing profession. It is in two parts: the first describes the complex organisational, social, historical, political and economic background to the research. The second part is an account of a three-year study of nurse management in one Regional Health Authority in the period 1985–8. The study describes the organisational changes that ensued after the introduction of general management following the Griffiths report (1983).

Nurses, like other health care professionals, are often sceptical about the role of management. The activities of managers are less visible than those in the clinical area. The outcomes are less obvious or immediately experienced than they are when patients are treated on an individual basis. It is not always clear what managers do in relation to the vigorous activity that accompanies patient care at the bedside, in the hospital or out in the community.

The management task of orchestrating financial, ideological and practical elements and moving them towards the same ends is complex, but central to good professional practice. The development of common policies, philosophies and values among health care workers is a necessary part of providing a service with high standards. But, often much that is said about good management seems mere rhetoric. The definitions of what constitutes good management, good standards and good policies are sometimes vague and incoherent.

Nevertheless, most of us know what we mean by a 'good service', especially if we become patients. Recently, a friend of one of the authors sat with her sister who was dying in a hospital. She was in great pain and begged to be relieved of her suffering. The nurses could not administer the necessary drugs without the doctor's permission, and the doctor was unable to attend. Consequently, this friend's sister died in agony.

Good management is an essential ingredient if the patient's needs are to be adequately met by a health service. Policies about care of the dying and administration of drugs have to be devised to make a service respond with humanity. What happens at the bedside may be the outcome of poor or ineffective management systems, or over-bureaucratic and authoritarian organisation.

Much emphasis in current NHS management is on financial and technical efficiency. To achieve this end, highly-skilled nurses and support workers are necessary. Finding the right balance in nursing care is itself a technical process, and cannot be divorced from issues of standards of care that can be measured and evaluated. This is a major management task.

Personal commitment of individual nurses and motivation at work are more abstract elements. However, these also need to be identified and nurtured. The nurse who is unable to control the pain of a dying patient because of unimaginative management policies will feel a failure. The primary task of managers of nurses is to help them to do their job well, to live up to the goals of the organisation, to care for patients within accepted and acceptable financial and technical parameters.

If management is well structured, and individuals are competent at their work, organisations and those who work in them will be capable of learning and adapting to new situations. We believe this book shows this complex learning process at work in a health service under great stress and undergoing profound changes. It is these positive aspects of high levels of professional and management commitment we should like to emphasise in this study.

Pat Owens
Howard Glennerster
September 1989

PART I

The Background

————————◆————————

Once problems are recognised ahead of time, they can easily be cured; but if you wait for them to present themselves, the medicine will be too late, for the disease will have become incurable.

(Machiavelli: *The Prince*, 1513)

1
The Griffiths prescription

—————— ◆ ——————

At present, the NHS is rather like a feudal society in which independent authority is exercised by a number of groups.... The Griffiths' proposals therefore imply as dramatic a transformation as that wrought by the Tudors after the Wars of the Roses.

(Day & Klein, 1983)

An important letter

On 6 October 1983, Roy Griffiths, deputy Chairman and Managing Director of Sainsbury's, wrote a letter to the Rt. Hon. Norman Fowler, MP, Secretary of State for Social Services. In 24 pages it set out the conclusions of his inquiry team on the managerial structure of the National Health Service (NHS), the largest employer in Britain. The team consisted of three other members – Mike Bett, Board Member for Personnel at British Telecom, Jim Blyth, Group Finance Director of United Biscuits and Sir Brian Bailey, Chairman of the Health Education Council. They were assisted by three civil servants. The team had only been appointed in February of the same year so it was, by the yardstick of government enquiries, a rapid piece of work. It began: 'This letter is not intended to be a major addition to the already considerable library of National Health Service literature'. Instead, it presented its recommendations in the form of 'management action to be taken by you'.

Despite this disarmingly unpretentious format, the letter contained proposals of radical nature and set in train potentially the most important internal reorganisation of the NHS since its creation in 1948. The central feature was the proposal to appoint general managers to run the Service. They would replace 'consensus' management teams that had been collectively responsible for taking decisions since 1974. Each of the new general managers would be responsible for a district unit of the NHS – a district hospital or all the community services in the area for example. The individuals would be the equivalent of the local manager of a Sainsbury's store. A single District General Manager (DGM) would be responsible for the whole service throughout a district.

Initially, the proposals were far from popular with professional groups within the Service. They made representation to MPs, and the House of Commons (1984) responded with a luke-warm report. It was the nursing organisations that were most critical. They saw the changes as a direct assault on their hard-won victories a decade earlier when nurses had gained representation at every decision-making level in the Service. The Royal College of Nursing launched a vigorous national advertising campaign to fight the changes in January 1986, but to no avail. Nurses have had to live with the changes and political attention has been diverted to wider issues of limited resources and increasing demands on the NHS *in general*. Nevertheless, the post-Griffiths changes have had major implications for nursing and have occurred at a critical time in the evolution of the profession in the UK.

This is a study of the way the Griffiths changes were implemented in one particular Health Service region, namely North West Thames. We concentrated on the implications that restructuring has had for the management of nursing service. Before proceeding, however, it is important to put the Griffiths recommendations into a longer-term perspective. A 24-page letter would never have had the impact that it did if it had not been addressing significant and long-standing problems within the NHS. We examine the origins of Griffiths diagnosis in the rest of this chapter.

The symptoms

The timing of Griffiths proposals was important. The founders of the Health Service had believed that rising living standards for the poor and a comprehensive free service that enabled everyone to get early treatment would *reduce* the demand for health care. In fact, as medical science improved and as people lived longer, the demands on the NHS increased. Moreover, the costs of meeting those demands grew faster than prices in the rest of the economy. In common with health care systems worldwide, the cost of health care was rising faster than the economy was growing. In the 1960s and early 1970s health spending rose twice as fast as the economy or personal incomes.

The oil crisis and the ensuing economic pressures produced a major reappraisal of the cost of health care. Governments in Britain and throughout the world began to try to contain and control health spending. It was not merely a matter of cost. There was also a growing suspicion that the professions and public sector unions had 'captured' the welfare state. It was they who were not responding to politicians reasonable requests, and were running the services in their own interests (Stewart & Shermon, 1967; Wilding, 1982).

However justified, these opinions found favour right across the political spectrum and were reflected in different governments' policies towards the NHS. The Labour Government in the mid 1970s had sought to achieve a shift in the spending priorities of the NHS by introducing cash limits to check the rise in spending. It sought to shift more resources to the care of the elderly, the mentally ill and handicapped, and to change the geographical distribution of spending. It found both tasks extremely difficult to achieve.

Ministers could *propose* but the complexity of local professional politics *disposed* (Glennerster, 1983). It proved very difficult to change spending patterns at local level. How were politicians to give the NHS direction? The Conservative administration came to power in 1979, committed to reducing public expenditure without endangering the standards of the social services. The NHS, in particular, would be 'safe' in their hands. The only way these apparently incompatible objectives could be achieved was to take refuge in the belief that the Health Service could achieve more by a more efficient use of its resources. That is what successive Ministers asked the Service to do (Ham, 1985).

From 1980–7 the real purchasing power of the money available to the hospital and community services in the NHS rose by only 0.5 per cent a year on average (Table 1.1) when prices and salary increases are taken into account. Thus the *real* additional resources available rose very slowly. Worse than that, the demands put upon

Table 1.1　*Resources and demands on the hospital and community services 1960–88 (percentage change per year)*

	Funds needed to meet demographic change	Actual increase in purchasing power per annum
1960–84	0.3	4.1
1981–82	0.4	1.9
1982–83	0.4	0.8
1983–84	0.5	0
1984–85	0.6	−0.1
1985–86	1.3	0.2
1986–87	1.0	0.5
1987–88	1.0	1.3

Source: *Health Finance: Assessing the Options* (King's Fund Institute, 1988); and *Financing and Delivering Health Care* (OECD, 1987) for 1960–84 figures.

the Health Service because of demographic change were rising at nearly double that rate.

In the year of the Griffiths Report and the following year, the real purchasing power available to the hospital and community services did not increase at all. If the politicians were to deliver their promises some 'magic' had to be performed. The efficiency of the Service had to increase dramatically, and some difficult choices had to be made. This was the essential problem Griffiths had to address but it was not a new one.

His report had been preceded by the Royal Commission on the NHS (1979), and the publication of the consultative paper 'Patients First' (DHSS, 1979). There had followed a major reorganisation of the management structure of the Service. The Area Health Authorities were removed and 192 new District Health Authorities (DHAs) were created, which were directly responsible to the Regional Health Authorities (RHAs). Moreover, power within the DHAs was delegated to the new units – local hospital or community services that were created as part of the 1982 reorganisation. The size of these 'units' varied between districts. During this period, savings on direct management costs were said to amount to £64m (Ham, 1985) but the upheaval had been considerable.

The diagnosis

Against this background it is not surprising to find several themes in Griffiths' letter.

1 *Direction*: The Service must be able to agree priorities. Therefore the Service needs 'leadership'.
2 *Economy*: The Service must be run with much greater attention to achieving value for money – 'cost improvement'.
3 *Accountability*: To do this requires clear lines of accountability of the professional staff to those who were responsible for managing the Service.
4 *Decentralisation*: These attributes can only be achieved by decentralising managerial responsibility.

Responding to the report soon after its publication, the late Tom Evans, Director of the King's Fund College argued that the essential 'spirit' of the report was 'the need to create a *managerial* culture in the NHS as opposed to what is still predominantly a professional and administrative culture'. The most quoted sentence in Roy Griffiths' letter summed up the problem as he saw it: 'In short, if Florence Nightingale were carrying her lamp through the corridors of the NHS today, she would almost certainly be searching for the people in charge' (para. 5). There was no one to give directions or to be held accountable for Health Service performance.

An inherited condition

This was not a new diagnosis. The condition had its origins in the pattern of medical care that had emerged in Britain long before the NHS was created. The NHS embodied three organisational forms, general practice, the local authority and the voluntary hospitals, that had developed over the previous century (Abel-Smith, 1964; Eckstein, 1958; Webster, 1988).

First, the family doctors or General Practitioners, had agreed to participate only as independent 'contractors'. The Family

Practitioner Committees that still oversee these services are independent authorities quite separate from the District Health
Authorities. No one can really be said to be 'in charge'.

The local authority

The second strand to the health care system used to be administered
by local authorities. It comprised the prevention of the spread of
infectious diseases, the long-stay hospitals and the provision of what
we today call the Community Health Services. These services were
all administered in a classical hierarchical fashion with a powerful,
high-profile figure at their head – the Medical Officer of Health,
who was a qualified doctor. He may have ranked low in the esteem
of the medical profession but he was an influential figure in the local
authority. He was a chief officer firmly in charge of his empire. In
1974, that separate empire finally disappeared to be amalgamated,
with the hospital services, into the new Health Authorities.

Some academic reformers with strong links with the public health
movement hoped that the Medical Officers, now transformed into
the new Community Physicians, would become the professional
leaders of the new service determining the needs of the area, setting
priorities, leading the planning process and giving the service
direction. It was always a flawed strategy (Lewis, 1987). The
medical officers never carried the prestige to outrank the senior
consultants in the acute sector. They had little experience of the
huge hospital sector that spent most of the money. The health
planning system never became the 'central lever of power' and this
left a power vacuum.

The voluntary hospitals

The traditions of the third health sector, the voluntary hospitals,
were to prove influential. They were an extraordinarily amorphous
group of institutions ranging from the large teaching hospitals to the
small local hospital. They had always been run with relatively weak
administrative and financial control and the medical profession
gained increasing power over the first decade of the Health Service.
The single hospital manager came to be replaced by the tripartite
consensus management team of the doctor, nurse and lay administrator (Murray, 1986). At regional level, administrative responsibility

was divided between the Senior Administrative Medical Officer and the Secretary to the Board, with no one officer being given precedence. From the outset, there were some who saw this lack of accountability as a major weakness in the new Health Service (Webster, 1988).

A say for nurses

It was against this background that the nursing profession began to press for the opportunity to be heard in the way that the doctors already were. Hospitals had become grouped together for administrative purposes. It had been found necessary to develop common nursing standards and procedures and to organise recruitment and training throughout the group. To that end, senior nursing posts were created but they were not part of any general career structure. A further problem was that Matrons, deputies and Ward Sisters created a system of 'triadic control', which confused lines of communication and accountability (Baly, 1973).

The Government was persuaded to appoint a committee of enquiry (Salmon Report, 1966), which recommended an extended range of posts in nursing management that lead from the Ward Sister up to that of a Chief Nursing Officer (CNO) – the pinnacle of the new structure, who was to act as a spokesperson for nurses and the head of the nursing service (Fig. 1.1).

The Mayston Report (1969) reflected the same logic as it applied to the local authority, or community nursing services as we call them today. Salmon reinforced the trend to the separate management and

Level of management	Rank	Grade
Top	Principal Nursing Officer Chief Nursing Officer	10 9
Middle	Nursing Officer (Matron) Senior Nursing Officer	8 7
First Line	Ward Sister/Charge Nurse Staff Nurse	6 5

Source: Armstrong (1981).

Figure 1.1   *The Salmon structure*

organisation of distinct occupational or professional groups within
the NHS, emulating the power hierarchy of the medical profession
and their independence. The Salmon report embodied the then
current practice of separate functional management very clearly.
The NHS was conceived as a coalition between exclusively managed
professional groups as if the NHS were a kind of marketplace in
which all the separate cottage industries plied their own trades.
Salmon put it more elegantly:

> The starting point is the patient, whose care or cure is the object
> of the enterprise and to this end many functions are discharged
> by many people working together. These should be managers of
> each major function – nursing, teaching, engineering,
> accounting and so on and their duty is to control their
> subordinates, that is to give them orders and coordinate their
> jobs.
>
> (para: 3:26)

Management by consensus

It was thought unnecessary for any one person or profession to be
in charge of the Health Service as a whole and that a process of
negotiation or discussion between professionals at the appropriate
level would resolve any conflicts. This belief reflected a change
in academic thinking about organisations. It put much more
emphasis on personal collaboration and less on authority structures
and formal bureaucratic hierarchies (Beatham, 1987). This view
was carried forward and embodied in the guidance set out by the
Department of Health and Social Security (1972) for the management of the new Health Authorities that were to run combined
hospital and community health services after 1974. The central
principle was expressed at the beginning of the 'Grey Book'
(DHSS, 1972) as it came to be called. It began by objecting to
the notion of putting one person in charge. The NHS was a complex
organisation and:

> Because of this complexity, organisation in a single hierarchy
> controlled by a chief executive is not appropriate. The
> appropriate structure is based on a unified management within
> the hierarchically organised professions, on representative

systems within the non-hierarchically organised medical and dental professions and on coordination *between* the professions. Coordination between professions at all levels will be achieved by multi-disciplinary teams through which the managers and representatives of the relevant professions can jointly make decisions.

(para. 1:24)

The teams will be consensus bodies, that is, decisions will need the agreement of each of the team members.

(para. 1:25)

Whatever may have been the merits of this organisational pre-scription in the relatively relaxed financial and political climate of the 1960s, it was ill-adapted to the financial climate of the 1980s. Although any manager will try to work in a climate of consensus where possible, harsh choices require someone to take the unpopular decision. Static or reduced budgets increase organisational conflict and the costs of change. They reduce organisations' capacity to take decisions on the basis of full consensus (Levine, 1978). Griffiths argued that attempts to reach consensus had lead to organisational inertia.

The cure – someone in charge!

The time was propitious for an old argument to re-emerge – the idea of a chief executive. Three decades before, the Bradbeer Committee (1954) had argued that efficient hospital administration required that one officer be charged with the responsibility to carry through the decisions of the hospital management boards and the policy of the Ministry of Health. This was also the view of a dissenting note to the Guillebaud Committee (1956), and the Farquharson-Lang Report (1966) in Scotland a decade later. That report argued for a Chief Executive in each hospital district.

The Labour Government's second Green Paper (DHSS, 1970) had advocated that the new unified Health Service should appoint a chief executive for each health authority, with a general manager at unit level to whom all professions and disciplines would be managerially accountable. This was reflected in the administrators' drive to gain more power and status within the Service. In her evidence to Sir Roy Griffiths, Mrs Kelly, the Chairman of the National Association of Health Authorities, returned to this old theme:

> The Chief Executive would have ultimate responsibility and be accountable to the authority for coordinating the whole exercise at district level – for developing a corporate plan, overseeing the implementation of policies and directing activities generally.
>   (NAHA Conference Report, 1983).

It was this model that Griffiths came to endorse.

The Griffiths model

At the centre in the Department of Health and Social Security there came to be a single multi-disciplinary NHS Management Board with a Chief Executive reporting to a Supervisory Board chaired by the Secretary of State (see Fig. 1.2 and discussion in Chapter 5). It gave a single set of directives to the Service replacing the multiple and separate systems of communication that had previously existed.

At regional and district level, a single individual, a general manager, should 'be charged with the general management function and overall responsibility for management's performance in achieving the objectives set by the authority' (para. 6:2). All day-to-day decisions should be taken 'in the main hospitals and other units of management' and while clinicians should be 'involved', management responsibility should be with a Unit General Manager with a single unit budget (paras 8:3 & 8:4). One person at each level, and most importantly at unit level, was to be in charge (see Fig. 1.2).

Further structural changes

In addition to these proposals, other suggestions were made in relation to management. These were limits to functional management, budgets for doctors, changes in the manager–professional relationship, power for the clinicians and a new personnel function.

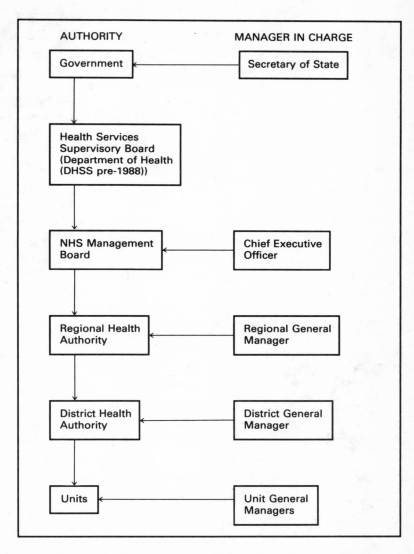

Figure 1.2   *The Post-Griffiths management structure for the NHS*

Limits to functional management

General management meant that the 'primary reporting relation-ship of the functional managers (like that of nursing managers) should be to the general manager'. Above the level of the unit, 'the relationship with the professions at other levels should simply be one of seeking guidance or monitoring the professional aspects of their work'. However, doctors in most districts in the country had professional accountability to their Regional Medical Officer (RMO) as contracts of employment were held regionally. So in practice, the District General Manager (DGM) was not, even in this new structure, to have total control.

Budgets for doctors

Each unit would develop a system of management budgets. It was proposed that each clinician would be allocated a budget that would cover all aspects of his or her activity. The resources of the hospital or service used would be costed out and attributed to that clinician. A budget ceiling would be set and the clinicians would not be able to spend above it (Griffiths, 1988 (para. 8:6)). This was, perhaps, the crux of the report and one on which some of those at the DHSS put most weight. It was the essential sanction general managers needed, if they were to contain medical costs and allocate priorities. As it turns out, it is the part of the proposed changes on which least progress has been made.

The manager–professional relationship

It was here that Griffiths (DHSS, 1984b) answered his own question 'will the general manager be in charge of professional staff?' thus:

> Taking a District General Manager as an example, he will be directly accountable to his DHA for the planning, implementation and control of performance. As such, he is responsible for ensuring that the professional staff have the opportunity of offering advice to the Authority. Once decisions have been taken, he will have the personal responsibility and authority for ensuring their implementation. Professional chief officers (for example, nursing advisers) will continue to be

directly accountable, and have right of access to the authority on the provision and quality of professional advice, but on matters relating to the general managers' responsibilities they will be accountable to him . . .

(p. 3)

If there is disagreement over a professional matter such as, for example, the level of pathology services necessary to support clinical works the doctor or other professional would be able to refer the matter to the Authority.

(p. 3)

The ultimate court of appeal thus lay beyond the general manager, at least in theory. There was to be a separate line of accountability for professional advice. No elucidation was given about such issues at unit level. Thus, right from the outset one crucial element in the role of general management, its precise relationship to the professions, remained open to various local interpretations.

Power for the clinicians – potential for conflict

There was a revealing section in the DHSS brief (DHSS, 1984b) dealing with doctors. It made it very clear that clinicians were 'clinically autonomous'. 'They are not responsible to any "top doctor", manager or even the Health Authority for their clinical decisions. The changes will in no way alter this position' (p. 4). The Authority was responsible for resources, however, and 'will therefore expect its general managers to be in regular discussions with consultants about the use of resources' (p. 4). There was no discussion of the nurse's position.

A new personnel function

It was not only general management that was given an enhanced role. Drawing again on the parallel with business, Personnel Directors were to be given a wider brief. The Central Management Board was to have a Personnel Director who would draw together matters of pay, performance, recruitment and career development. The implication was that similar posts should be created at lower levels in the service. References were made to the analysis of manpower needs and determination of optimum levels for nursing manpower (p. 8).

Nurses' reactions

The medical professions reacted in a rather guarded way to the proposed changes (*Brit.Med.J.*, Editorial, June 1984). But the failure to include the Chief Nursing Officers at the DHSS on the Supervisory Board set up by Griffiths caused 'dismay and resentment', and was seen as a deliberate attack on the profession. The Social Services Committee Report (House of Commons, 1984) hastily recommended that this state of affairs was revised.

The Royal College of Nursing (RCN), in particular, had been influential in creating the framework of senior management posts in nursing that followed the Salmon Report. It saw very quickly that Griffiths had major implications for senior nurse managers and the potential for destroying this structure. Hitherto, there had been a nursing officer on the consensus management team at each level in the service. Chief Nursing Officers, at district or regional levels, and their staff were line managers operating above the unit level and they were liable to be swept away. Unified unit budgets meant the loss of the CNO's separate budget-holding responsibility for nurse manpower in the districts. The enhanced personnel function would mean a loss of responsibility by nurses for nurse staffing.

Managerial responsibility for nurses at levels above the unit would be lost, being replaced by an 'advisory function'. What would happen at unit level was unclear. It was feared that nurses could lose all control over nursing staff here too. The RCN was particularly critical of the appointment of Unit General Managers (UGMs), which they saw most in conflict with the hitherto explicit nurse managers' responsibility for the nursing workforce (*Nursing Mirror*, Editorials, 1983).

Critical evidence was subsequently given to the House of Commons Social Services Committee and received a sympathetic hearing. The Committee recommended that a nurse be a member of the Supervisory Board and that the Government give more thought to the creation of Unit General Managers (House of Commons, 1984). It soon became clear, however, that the Government was going to press ahead with Griffiths' recommendations (DHSS, 1984b).

The RCN therefore took the unprecedented step of mounting a national advertising campaign in the press in January 1986, opposing the changes as they would affect nursing. It began with a picture of Florence Nightingale alongside a modern nurse. The caption read, 'The nurse on the left established British nursing standards. The nurse on the right is being forced to compromise them.' (*The Times*, 12.1.86.)

This was followed by another advertisement showing a general manager pictured with a calculator and the caption, 'Why is Britain being run by people who do not know their *coccyx* from their *humerus*?' (*The Times*, 14.1.86) Another advertisement pictured a nursing sister and said, 'She has great faith in the NHS, which is more than the NHS has in her'. (*Guardian*, 21.1.86.) The thrust of all three advertisements was that nurses were best qualified to run nursing, that Directors of Nursing Services (DNSs) should be present in all units, as they were already, and that nurses should not be excluded from important decision-making processes and relegated to an advisory role without the 'power . . . to make health care more effective'. Each advertisement had a small form that could be filled in and sent off stating: 'I agree that nursing should be run by nurses.'

According to Alison Dunn, Director of Press and Publicity at the RCN, proposals for reorganisation at Unit level, which also did away with the Director of Nursing Services and threatened all nurse managers above the Ward Sister were particularly worrying (Dunn, 1986). The advertising campaign was attempting to influence the structures that were just beginning to emerge as new District General Managers and unit managers were appointed. It was a projection of an image of nurses as 'the patient's friend' and advocate. At the same time, it was an expression of the anxiety felt by the profession about losing power within the NHS.

Images and reality

This advertising campaign was in progress while we were conducting our first round of interviews both with senior nurses and with the new general managers, described in Part II. It is worth pausing to reflect on the advertisements themselves, briefly, as the images that were projected to the public were far from accidental, they were carefully chosen to send messages about the profession's self-perceptions.

The conflict centred around the concept of 'advice' and 'management' and the idea that in the new organisation nurses would be without *power* and relegated to a passive advisory role to management. The memory of Miss Nightingale was called upon in the quest to save nursing standards. Emotive language was used, '. . . a matter of life and death can become a matter of pounds and pence'. This suggested that the new managers were more interested in balancing the books than caring for patients.

In the advertisements, the general manager was portrayed as a man, the pocket calculator being a symbol of his new role – the quest for cost-effectiveness. The suggestion was that he would exclude nurses from important areas of management where their expertise was needed. The image was of the traditional nurse complete with uniform, frilly cap and clip-board, and of the profession's ancestor Florence Nightingale who symbolised the ethic of service that was being phased out by the changes Griffiths had recommended.

Nurses face uncertainty

No organisational blueprint was proposed in the Griffiths Report. The main emphasis was on making the doctors both clinically and financially responsible and developing clear lines of accountability to the ultimate authority of the general manager. It was uncertain how this would work out in practice for the nurses, but this issue of professional accountability to a manager who was not a nurse was the first question to be raised.

The other principal theme, that of making the Service more efficient and cost-effective, also had ramifications for nurses. It was suggested that the management structure was top heavy, and that nurse manpower levels needed reassessment. This created major anxieties among the nurses in management who feared losing their jobs, and having their qualified staff replaced by cheaper, unskilled workers. On both counts, the report was viewed as a threat – a dilution of the power, importance and value of nurses in the NHS.

Organisational change had preceded Griffiths' letter, but it was a transformation that continued at an accelerated pace after 1984, when his recommendations were implemented. The psychological effects of such drastic change on those working in the NHS cannot be overestimated. Reorganisation for many managers had meant seeing their colleagues phased out, or having to compete for their own jobs, or for fewer jobs. To some extent it explained a certain reluctance to undergo further change (Carrier & Kendal, 1986).

Although Griffiths had not recommended further reorganisation, this did not quite equate to some of the other suggestions he was making. Reducing levels of staff in management, the introduction of general management above the levels necessary for functional management, and stringent cost-effectiveness drives made it seem inevitable that some restructuring would occur.

Even in situations where general managers preferred to leave their staff in relative peace, the future remained uncertain. What Griffiths had done was to open the door to endless possibilities, to raise the issue of change as a permanent feature of the Health Service's continuous need to adapt to external pressures in the face of rapid social and technological change.

At the same time, nursing had reached a crossroads. It was experiencing growing staffing difficulties. It was faced with a crisis of professional identity when the educational needs of nurses had not kept pace with sociological and technological change. Most of all, it was faced with a crisis of meaning in terms of nurses' place and value in modern society, and within our health care system today.

2

Nursing troubles: the external environment

—————— ◆ ——————

The major changes that have taken place in nursing have been part of a turbulent National Health Service. The experiences we recount in Part Two cannot really be understood outside that context. The essential argument of this chapter is that the task of managing, leading and supporting nurses at every level in the Service has grown more demanding, just at the point when substantial changes were taking place in the organisation of those who were to undertake these tasks.

The great funding debate

Throughout this period was a growing debate about the funding of the National Health Service, which lead, in 1988, to a major Prime Ministerial review. Nursing was at the heart of that debate. First, nursing salaries are an important element in the cost of the NHS. In 1987–8 nurses salaries cost £4364m, accounting for 22 per cent of the NHS budget (Review Body, 1988). Second, their pay has had to rise faster than other costs. In 1984, nurses were awarded a 7.5 per cent rise, which added £216 million to the NHS budget over and above the 3 per cent already allowed for pay increases. Although Central Government found most of the extra sum, £36m had to come from 'efficiency' savings in the Service as a whole. Thus the success of nurses in winning pay awards from the independent review body put strains on the rest of the Service.

In 1985, a group representing the doctors, nurses and general managers produced a joint report that argued that little additional efficiency savings could be made (NIHSM, BMA & RCN, 1985). They were supported by the House of Commons Social Services

Committee (House of Commons, 1986). The MPs argued that an immediate 2 per cent increase in cash was needed to sustain existing standards of care and that pay awards should be fully funded by the Government. The DHSS did not agree and asserted that general managers should be able to improve effectiveness still further (DHSS, 1986).

By late 1986, an air of defeat had crept into the comments on NHS funding. The extra £700m promised by the Chancellor was seen to be a drop in the ocean. Day & Klein (1986) wrote that the recognition that the NHS was underfunded and probably would continue to be, 'can lead to a downward spiral in which declining morale leads to the development of defensive organisational attitudes which, in turn, breed a sense of defeat'.

In the autumn and winter of 1987–8, a series of well-publicised personal stories put health service resources on the political agenda once again and nursing featured in them all. The cases of children with cardiac problems having to wait too long for operations were highlighted, and shortages of essential Intensive Care Unit (ICU) nurses was one reason for the postponement of operations (*The Times*, Seton, 1987b). One parent brought a case against the DHA applying for a judicial review of the Health Authority's failure to allocate funds, but the Court of Appeal refused permission (Law Report, *The Times*, 1987).

By the beginning of 1988, the Cabinet were showing signs of dissatisfaction at the handling of the NHS funding crisis (Webster, 1988). There were dramatic scenes in the Commons when an Opposition MP was suspended for interrupting prayers accusing the Government of 'inhuman' health policies. The uproar was caused by newspaper reports about the time that babies and children were waiting for heart operations (Seton, 1987a; Seton, 1987b; Veitch, 1987b).

This whole series of events was to have an unsettling effect on nurses and managers alike. Nursing had moved to the centre of political debate.

Nursing recruitment and national politics

Although local managers and educators had been aware of the problem for a long time, the recruitment and retention of nursing staff became a national issue in the mid 1980s. From 1981–2 to 1986–7, the numbers entering basic training fell by 29 per cent. Of those accepted for training, 21 per cent failed to qualify or register, or work in the NHS (Price-Waterhouse, 1988); this happened despite improvements in pay and hours of work.

The most important reason for this was a sharp fall in the size of the age group who normally become nurses. The total number of school leavers, and hence the normal pool for recruitment, peaked in 1984–5 but fell steadily after that, and would probably fall by about a quarter by 1994. The NHS would soon need to recruit around a third of the girls in this group to meet its needs for nurses (Committee of Public Accounts, 1987). In addition, a substantial number of nurses were beginning to join the private sector – Delamothe, (1988) suggests at a rate of up to 1000 a year. Also the demographic trend towards an increasingly elderly population was putting greater demands on the nursing service just as nursing supply began to decline.

Pay has been another factor influencing the current crisis. Since 1979, the pay of Staff Nurses has increased by 34 per cent in real terms. But in spite of this, they have lagged behind salaries young people could command in the more prosperous cities. As nursing is still a female-dominated profession, gender is one explanation for the persistence of low pay. In other public services that are predominantly male, such as the police and fire services, *starting* salaries are comparable with those earned by qualified nurses after eight or nine years. Forty per cent of nurses earn less than the Low Pay Unit's threshold (Delamothe, 1988).

The National Union of Public Employees published a survey that claimed that in seven out of ten nursing households their pay made up nearly half of the total household income, and that about one third of all nurses had three or more children living at home (NUPE and LPU, 1987). There is some evidence that a high proportion of nurses head one-parent families, and are therefore wholly dependent on their pay (Delamothe, 1988).

The *British Medical Journal* ran a series of articles about nursing, the first of which began, 'Who would have thought even a year ago that when the crunch came in the National Health Service it would have come with nurses?' (Delamothe, 1988). Many observers would not have been so surprised. The nursing unions had been pressing for a major package of changes, not merely higher pay but educational reform, a better working environment, more supportive management, the provision of child care facilities, better differential career prospects, and more mature students with special entrance requirements (Hildrew, 1987a).

The Fifth Report of the Review Body for Nursing Staff (1988) endorsed much of this case. In 1987, Regional Health Authority Chairmen reported on a study of nursing vacancies. Overall, 3.5 per cent of funded posts had been vacant for more than 3 months compared with 3.2 per cent in the previous year. Some vacancy rates had risen faster, for example District Nurses and Health Visitors. Over 40 per cent of vacancies were for Staff Nurses. Midwifery and special care baby units were among those with the highest vacancy rates. The London area was worst of all – vacancy rates of 20 per cent were found in inner London. Difficulties were particularly severe in the Thames regions with high turnover rates, substantial falls in the numbers entering training and high wastage rates during training were among factors mentioned (para. 20).

> One district had interviewed leavers between May and September 1987 and had found that two thirds of them were Staff Nurses, that nearly 40 per cent of them were leaving NHS work altogether and that most of them who were staying in the NHS were moving away from London. The factors said to have influenced their decisions to leave were: low pay (the deciding factor for two thirds of those leaving the NHS); low status; long hours/shift work; and general lack of concern for nursing as a profession. Other factors included poor accommodation, inadequate support services and weak management.
>
> (para. 21)

A separate submission from District Chairmen in North West Thames argued that special factors in the South East, especially pay and living costs, were creating acute shortages and flexible pay arrangements were necessary. Nurses were leaving for better paid jobs in the private sector. In inner London, average gross earnings for a Staff Nurse were 16 per cent below the regional average for female non-manual earnings.

The Review Body finally offered an overall rise in salary of 15.3 per cent, but this figure concealed the fact that some nurses would receive up to 60 per cent and others as low as 4 per cent. Jobs were to be regraded, reflecting 'the biggest restructuring of staff in the health industry for 40 years'. It had been suggested that there should be flexible local pay arrangements but this was rejected by the Review Body (Sherman, 1988c). Some areas were identified as having special problems with recruitment because of housing and transport costs in inner London and the periphery, East Anglia, Oxford and Wessex Regions. Nevertheless, the unions have continued to resist further pressure to give additional weightings to certain areas. The RCN warned of 'turbulence of a high order' (Sherman, 1988e).

The pay award was to be funded in full by the Government, and not, as in the past, partially subsidised by DHAs already over-stretched financially. However, in August 1988, the grading pay structure ran into trouble because of the insistence that, on each ward, only one Sister would be eligible for the highest pay award. Consequently, a day of protest was organised by COHSE. The main action was at the Middlesex Hospital where 55 nurses arranged a 24-hour strike; smaller actions took place elsewhere.

By October 1988, and after further talks with regional Chairmen, the Government agreed that the pay award had been underfunded, and that further money would be found to meet the anomalies in the grading structure. The National Association of Health Authorities (NAHA) suggested that additional funds of about £150m over and above the original £803m would be necessary to meet the cost of the clinical gradings. Anxiety was growing in the DHAs that the figures that the Government was using were inaccurate. In response to these pressures and union unrest, the Secretary of State agreed that the Government would meet fully the estimated shortfall in funding of around £100m (Sherman, 1988d).

Union militancy and conflict

A new militancy among nurses had emerged in the three years of this study and a more open divide between the RCN and the other unions COHSE and NUPE. Jane Salvage, author of *The Politics of Nursing* (1985), suggests that the new radicalism is, in part, a response to the new tougher management style nurses are finding in their units. Managers with limited budgets and encouragement 'to be tough' are faced in return with a more militant workforce and hostile unions, which in turn makes management more difficult.

In the US, exactly the same financial pressures have produced similar tensions. Hospital managers are looking for cheaper workers to do the nurses' tasks. Nurses feel 'threatened from below' as less-trained workers are hired (Melosh, 1986). In Britain, the nursing unions showed they had the potential power to either defend or threaten the stability of the Service. Still retaining public support, unlike other unions, they exerted unexpected leverage in the battle for funds.

Deeper forces at work

Thus in 1988, nurses were scarcely out of the national newspapers for a week at a time. Shortages of highly skilled staff in all areas, serious shortages of all grades of staff in some places, pay, regrading, recruitment and retention of staff had all become political issues. Headlines ran: 'The nursing scandal' (Hildrew, 1987a), 'Nurses offered new deal' (Hildrew, 1987b), 'Bitter row as Thatcher hits NHS strike' (Oakley, 1988), 'Government's aim is a free nurses' market' (Sherman, 1988a), 'Nurses in RCN warned against joining strikes' (Gapper, 1988), 'Government move to diffuse nursing pay crisis' (Sherman, 1988d).

In order to understand why this should have occurred we must look beyond the issues of pay and difficulty with grading. These are merely symptoms of deeper changes in society and health care that are also to be found in other countries, notably in the USA, despite its very different form of finance and administration. Figure 2.1 illustrates the complexity of forces at work in addition to the internal crisis in nursing and the disputes over pay. There are not only financial and demographic pressures, but also public and political pressures.

Financial constraints

These are not unique to the UK (OECD, 1987) but here they are more tightly drawn. Advanced industrialised countries spend, on average, 7.5 per cent of their incomes on health care. The UK figure is 5.9, and ranks among the lowest in the Western world. Many other European countries spend far more, and the figure for the US is about 11 per cent. The gap between the professions' technical

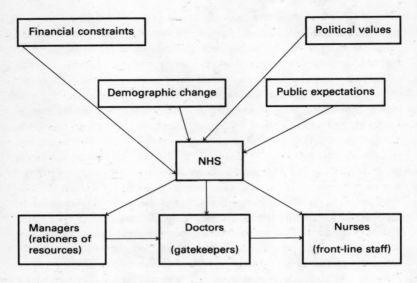

Figure 2.1 *The external environment*

capacity to care, and their actual capacity to do so, is thus wider in the UK than in most other countries. The fact that many wasteful procedures are avoided in this country is economically good, but it imposes a far greater burden on the manager. He or she has to act as a 'rationer' of resources – the person who has to say 'no'.

Demographic pressure

The elderly are the major users of the Health Service. The most rapidly rising age group are the over 80s and health needs rise exponentially with age. The needs of a 60-year-old are several times greater than those of a person in his or her 20s and those of an 80-year-old between five and ten times those of a 60-year-old (Craig, 1983). The psychological demands on staff are particularly significant, complete recovery and 'success' are less easy to gain in old age.

Public expectations

These are even more powerful sources of external pressure. Medical science has been ascribed almost magical powers. Medicine, as

Illich (1977) has put it, has come to be seen as a defence against death. Death outside old age is seen as unnatural and preventable. Blame is to be attached if it occurs, and doctors and nurses are seen to have failed. Natural death, we think, comes in old age and has come to be seen almost as a civil right.

Other writers such as Gorer (1965), Levine & Scotch (1970), and Ariès (1976) have suggested that death has become a process that has had to be 'hushed up'. 'One no longer dies at home in the bosom of one's family, but in hospital alone; and one dies in hospital because the doctors did not succeed in healing.' Death has become a technical phenomenon that happened because care ceased, and was often the decision of the doctor and hospital team (Glaser & Strauss, 1979).

Modern death has therefore become medicalised. Death will, in all probability, be dealt with by doctors and nurses. There has been a shift of responsibility by the public onto professionals in the health services who are often young, inexperienced and overworked. In a more general context, death has become almost a taboo subject (Gorer, 1965). In advanced industrial cultures, there is a denial of death (Kellehear, 1984). It is within this culture that modern medicine is functioning and trying to make choices.

The life-prolonging activities of doctors has its effect on nurses who take on the outcomes of treatments, which increase the daily workload. These techniques make greater demands for higher levels of technical skill in nursing to perform treatments. They also place higher emotional strains on staff dealing with people who are chronically sick and highly dependent. Nationally, 60–75% of all deaths occur within an institution (NWTRHA, 1987).

Political values

For those working in the National Health Service such pressures were not new. They had partially been offset by the high degree of public support the service received, which gave their work a high social worth. There was a basic satisfaction to be gained by being part of one of the most valued social institutions in the country. However, as the 1980s advanced, they saw that degree of political support eroding. Public services in general were not well regarded. The political consensus that the NHS was the best vehicle for health care and something to be proud of began to erode. The service was a 'state monopoly', 'over bureaucratic', and as a State Service dependent on taxation it would continue to be underfunded. The private market was extolled. The Service was in 'terminal decline' and radical new measures were needed for private funding and provision (Pirie & Butler, 1988; Peet, 1987; Goldsmith & Willetts, 1988; Letwin & Redwood, 1988).

Some thought that the Government was deliberately setting out to destabilise the Service by asking it to fund pay awards agreed by politicians nationally, and by setting more than a score of so-called 'priorities', which were, in total, unrealistic. This change in the political climate and the ensuing depression and psychological effect it was having on those who worked in the Service is impossible to measure or 'prove', but it was expressed by many in the NHS during the research.

The cascade effect

Under the new Griffiths structures, it was the general managers who were explicitly given the task of resolving these contradictory pressures. They were to ensure that the Service worked within the limits set by Government. They were now the rationers of resources, but not the gatekeepers of the Service, as the doctors still had the clinical freedom that Griffiths endorsed. It is the clinicians who decide whom and how many to refer to hospitals for treatment, whom and how many shall be admitted and what treatment to give for how long.

It is the manager's task to negotiate the basic resource a hospital doctor has, such as the number of beds in a specialty. Yet, in the traditional British system, all the other resources a doctor uses are free. If a consultant admits more patients and treats them more quickly, increased numbers of patients can pass through the same number of beds. This puts more demand on the support services, drugs, theatre costs and nurses.

Doctors in Birmingham who had increased their own productivity were asked to reduce their workloads by 10 per cent (Timmins & Spackman, 1987) because it was increasing other costs. Thus attempts to constrain budgets in the face of rising demands involve a long chain of consequences. Managers must negotiate with doctors about bed space and ward facilities, assessing the impact of admissions and treatment schemes on other services and costs. Nurses and junior medical staff are profoundly affected by these processes. No one wants their unit or their clinical team not to respond to the expectations the public have of the service. The pressure is to do increasingly more with the same resources; thus the consequent pressures and demands tend to be passed down to the weaker staff members. This, in turn, has tended to produce increased militancy and ambivalence among nurses. These conflicts were played out on a national stage.

Politicians' response to such an analysis is to point to the substantial increases that have taken place in the numbers of nursing staff. Moores (1987) analysed the trends in British hospitals between 1962 and 1984. Over that period, the whole time equivalent (WTE) number of staff rose by nearly half (47 per cent). Yet the basic hours worked by each fell. The working week was shortened from 44 hours in 1968 to 37.5 in 1984. An extra week's holiday and other bank holiday provisions further reduced the hours worked. Each nurse thus worked a fifth fewer hours. Conversely, inpatient cases rose by 46 per cent and the average length of stay fell by nearly half. That was enough, Moores claims, to increase the workload by 32 per cent. In short, the increase in staffing had been offset by the scale and intensity of care being provided. Indeed, this is a process that has gone on since the nineteenth century (Abel-Smith, 1962).

Summary

Nurses became one of the most sensitive political groups during the period of the study, which was reflected in the importance that general managers began to give to nursing issues. The tasks of management in the NHS grew more difficult in the period that followed the Griffiths report for reasons unconnected with that report. This was especially true of nursing. Changing social expectations, political values and financial constraints put great strains on a large, youthful workforce at a time when other better-paid job opportunities were developing fast in the service economy (Nicholson-Lord, 1988). Nursing was at a disadvantage in competing for a declining absolute number of young people in the age group that usually entered nursing, although it was still a popular option among girls. The external pressures added to an internal debate about the future of nursing, which had its origins in the birth and historical development of the profession, as described in the following chapter.

3
Nursing troubles: internal tensions

———————— ◆ ————————

Just as one set of external pressures were putting an increasing strain on the Health Service, and hence on nurses, so a different set of social forces were causing tensions within nursing itself. Clashes of values and interest were being fought out. We illustrate these tensions in Figure 3.1. Few were new but several took on greater significance during the period of our field work. Together these conflicts complicated professional and managerial relationships at every level.

```
Exclusive profession <------> Extensive workforce
Profession            <------> Trade union
Pure nursing          <------> General management responsibilities
Holistic practice     <------> Specialist practice
Senior clinicians     <------> Senior managers
Female                <------> Male
```

Figure 3.1 *Nursing contradictions*

A divided ancestry

How do groups hold together over time and carry forward their values from one generation to another? Anthropologists suggest that the most powerful vehicles are myth (Malinowski, 1974; Lévi-Strauss, 1977) and ritual (Van Gennep, 1960). Conceptions of the past and activities of the present are usually associated with some explanation about the genesis of the group, and the genitor. Usually, ancestors epitomise the principal ideologies that the group holds corporately, they symbolise the structure of that collectivity. By tracing descent from a particular ancestor, descendents can validate the claims of property rights or more general morality in terms of a definable past (Douglas, 1987).

Nursing, as we know it today, has *several* ancestries that represent competing values and ideals. The figure in the Vatican of the goddess Hygeia serving the physician Asklepios is an early depiction of the subservient relationship of women to men in the healing process (Nutting & Dock, 1907). Yet during the early Christian and Medieval periods, both men and women in religious orders nursed the sick or performed as physicians. A tradition of admirable women, possessing intellect, prudence and common sense was characteristic of the early ancestors of nursing.

The most potent figure of this kind in nursing history in Britain is surely Florence Nightingale, at whose door much praise and blame has been placed. She, above all, is the natural symbol of one set of nursing values, and the guardian of group solidarity and morality. Every year a lamp is ritually carried to Westminster Abbey to commemorate this ancestor and reaffirm group values. Florence Nightingale defined the practice of nursing, and the myths that surround her provide contradictory images of a gentle, angelic figure and dominant powerful leader. However, there is a separate heritage in nursing, that of militant trade unionism, which emerged not from the voluntary hospitals but from the asylums and Poor Law institutions.

The Nightingale myth is both revered and criticised, nurtured and rejected. Nurses today simultaneously seek to emulate and denigrate her image as they attempt to reconcile the past of professionalism *and* trade union militancy in the present.

The quest for respectability

Nurses in the middle of the nineteenth century came from the servant or domestic class, or were recruited from the paupers in the workhouse. Nurse training was either non-existent, or haphazard depending on the standards of the institutions in which they worked. As *The Times* put it in 1857, nurses were:

> Lectured by committees, preached at by chaplains, scowled at by treasurers and stewards, scolded by matrons, sworn at by surgeons, bullied by dressers, grumbled at and abused by patients, insulted if old and ill-favoured, talked flippantly to if middle-aged and good-humoured, tempted and seduced if young and well-looking, they are what any woman might be under these circumstances.

(Abel-Smith, 1960)

Modern student nurses are taught that the reform of nursing can be traced back to the foundation of the Nightingale School in 1860 at St. Thomas' Hospital. Two types of recruits were trained, 'ladies' who paid for themselves and ordinary probationers who were maintained. But the higher social class of many of the women meant that doctors feared that their authority would be undermined. Consequently, the School itself was not opened without considerable opposition from hospital doctors. One surgeon remarked that these ladies would never be content until they had become the executives of the hospitals, as they had already done in the army, and 'had been a constant source of annoyance to medical and surgical officers' (Abel-Smith, 1960).

The case for registration, and opposition to it, caused a schism in the ranks of nursing. Ethel Bedford-Fenwick, the protagonist for registration, stated that 'the nurse question is the woman question'. The new 'lady' nurses were seeking to enhance their status, and wanted parity with the medical profession. She was anxious to give nurses autonomy and value in society, to provide them with an education, which would engender confidence and independence and give status.

Florence Nightingale opposed registration on the grounds that personal qualities were of the foremost importance in selecting and training a nurse. Hospital managers who opposed the Nurses' Registration Act of 1919 feared that it would restrict the supply of nurses and tend to raise their pay. The regulations that insisted on living-in training reduced the number of elderly widows and married women in the profession. Consequently, the average age of nurses fell and the loss of older women contributed to growing shortages.

Throughout the 1920s and 1930s these shortages continued and became a permanent feature of the Service. Then, as now, a large part of care was actually undertaken by un-registered nurses. This was partly because developments in medicine made increasing demands for nursing care. The greater demands of war also lead to the 1943 Nurses Act, which created a second grade of nurse, the State Enrolled Nurse (SEN), despite the vigorous opposition of many leaders of the profession it was supported by the trade unions (Abel-Smith, 1960).

The registered nurses were always at pains to distance themselves from the unqualified in their ranks and, consequently, over the years a kind of caste system within the Service has developed. It extends from the senior nurse/generalists at one end of the spectrum to the unqualified nurse at the other with numerous sub-strata in between, all struggling for status and respectability.

The profession continued to act as if there were an endless supply of 'ladies' to fill the qualified nursing role. *It was never so in the past* despite the Nightingale myth. At present, the career options for the same educated women that the nursing profession wishes to attract are so much wider that only a relatively modest proportion of them can be expected to enter the profession.

The history of nursing is therefore a consistent failure by the leaders of the profession to face this reality. The division between the ancestors, Mrs Bedford-Fenwick and Florence Nightingale in the past, and the RCN and the NHS unions today, has prevented the profession from speaking with one voice, and from finding a consensus about the 'nature' of nursing, which encompasses its plurality.

The tenacity and will of nursing leaders to develop standards and stick by them in the face of falling numbers of recruits is admirable, and it is this idealism that has consistently carried the profession forward. But too tenacious a hold on principles may in the long run be a destructive force. Dunea, writing of the American experience in 1988, remarks that we live in 'an age obsessed with classroom education'. The nursing profession in the USA has constantly upgraded its educational requirements. Promotion now depends to a large extent on educational qualifications, which, he contends, leads to overqualification. Consequently, the clinically-oriented nurse reaches a dead end, or ends up in administration.

Nursing leaders have continually pressed for more professional nurses and fewer skilled aids on the wards. In response to the economic crisis of recent years, 'embattled hospitals went half way by buying off the practical nurses and nursing aids ... leaving "the nurse" alone ... a general without an army' (Dunea, 1988).

In Britain, the need for qualified nurses is now generally accepted and the respect accorded to nurses as professionals is openly acknowledged, but at the same time the continued contribution made by unqualified staff given less attention.

This fundamental dilemma has never been fully resolved. Should nurses strive for high professional status, longer training and greater exclusivity following the model of the medical profession? Does nursing require large numbers of staff with less in the way of formal education to undertake important caring duties? If the Health Service actually requires *both*, what is to be the relationship and balance between these two kinds of nursing staff? The more restrictive the financial climate, the greater the strains between these two philosophies.

During the period of this research, nursing education and training once more came under review while addressing these problems.

In 1986, the UK Central Council for Nursing, Midwifery and Health Visiting published its proposals for a complete recasting of nurses' training – *Project 2000: A New Preparation for Practice* (UKCC, 1986). In 1988 the Government gave its broad support to these proposals. The new educational institutions would be independent from Service delivery and have close links with higher educational institutions outside nursing. Trainees would be given student status and would be supernumerary to the nursing establishment during their three-year course. They would receive student grants, not pay. About a fifth of their time would be counted as a Service contribution. The proposals envisaged 3 kinds of nurse: 'The *registered practitioner* would be competent to assess the need for care, to provide that care, to monitor and to evaluate care and to do all this in a range of institutional and non institutional settings' (para: 5.14).

Above the registered practitioner would be several kinds of *specialist* practitioner who would have direct care responsibilities but be able to give advice and support to the registered practitioners. Below the registered nurse would be the *aide* or support worker, directly supervised and monitored by the registered practitioner.

These potential changes, of course, affected the way senior nurses, in particular, viewed the organisational changes that were taking place in the service. They made the planning of nursing education and its relationship with service delivery an absolutely crucial issue. It would require careful thought at both district and regional level.

Nurse specialist or general manager?

Another argument of long standing is the extent to which senior nurses should concern themselves with the supervision of nurses alone or whether nursing encompasses the whole environment within which nurses work.

The Nightingale myth, 'the gentle vision of female virtue' (Strachey, 1918) was, in reality, a potent driving force that re-organised the kitchen and launderies in army hospitals, supervised the building of wards, their ventilation, drains and sewers and supplies of medicine, beds and clothing. In her own words, nursing was 'the least important of the functions into which one had been forced'. Lytton Strachey wrote, 'she filled papers with recommendations and suggestions, with criticisms of the minutist details of organisation, with elaborate calculations of contingencies, with exhaustive analyses and statistical statements piled up in breathless eagerness one on top of the other'. She criticised incompetent doctors or self-sufficient nurses, and her attacks on unbending and inert officialdom had 'the deadly and unrelenting precision of a machine-gun' (Strachey, 1918).

Such a description could well be applied to some contemporary general managers in the NHS. The fact that Florence Nightingale perceived nursing as an essentially female occupation did not mean that she accepted the idea of 'women's work' and 'men's work' as mutually exclusive. In *Notes on Nursing*, published in 1859, she wrote: 'Keep clear of the jargon which urges women to do nothing that men do, merely because they are women . . .' and because 'this is women's work' and 'that is men's', and 'these are things that women should not do . . . which is all assertion and nothing more . . . . You want to do the thing that is good whether it is suitable for a woman or not.'

The Matron, like her domestic housekeeper equivalent in Victorian England, ran the whole household economy, including the domestics and the kitchen staff. But the profession in the twentieth century moved increasingly towards a medical model of training and to a purely nursing function. This professional ideal was expressed most clearly in the Salmon Report in the 1960s and also in the reorganisation that followed, which set up a pure nursing hierarchy managed separately from other occupational groups. Many nurses, holding an alternative vision of nursing, objected to these moves at the time as they held to older more all-embracing traditions (Briggs, 1972).

These contrary ancestries help to explain the ambivalence nurses had in responding to the extended roles that many general managers were pressing on them in the 1980s. The general managers wanted nurses to take on extended general management roles, being responsible not just for the nurses on a ward but all the staff. But nurses were reluctant to relinquish the power inherent in the hierarchy of the Salmon structure, which gave senior nurses managerial parity with senior doctors and administrators.

Other contradictions existed at the bedside level. Student nurses are taught the importance of seeing each patient as a complete person, of assessing their needs, determining the appropriate kind of care and following that patient through all their stages by using Individual Care Plans (ICPs). Once again the principle lies deep in the nursing myth. In practice, a nurse on the modern ward often finds the pressures and the speed of turnover so great that such a process is frequently impossible to follow (Melia, 1987).

Much of the day-to-day care in many hospitals, especially long-stay hospitals, is undertaken by unregistered nurses who have little or no training. About 50 per cent of all care is given by unregistered nurses particularly in the mental handicap and elderly sectors. At the same time, the need for highly trained and specialised nurses is growing as the specialised nature of medicine grows. Here the interests of educators, practitioners and service managers are often difficult to reconcile.

Militant angels?

If the struggle to turn nursing into a profession belongs to its history with its own traditions and values, so too does the history of militant trade unionism (Carpenter, 1982; Salvage, 1985). Nurses in the long-stay Poor Law hospitals were very poorly paid. There was always a supply of paupers who could be recruited. Conditions of pay were also bad for those who worked in the asylums. It was they who joined the National Asylum Workers Union that organised a series of strikes after the First World War. Even in the 1920s the College of Nursing was opposing the strike weapon as 'unprofessional'.

It was after the Second World War, in 1946, that the Poor Law workers and the asylum workers amalgamated to form the Confederation of Health Service Employees (COHSE). As the size of the work force grew and became more specialised and hierarchical and as hospitals became rather more like industrial enterprises, so trade unionism grew. Even the RCN has adopted more militant postures. It has a high representation on the Whitley Councils and has developed a 'steward' structure.

Some nurse managers saw many of their problems as a reflection of the competition between the unions for members. There was also a profound clash of values. For example some nurses responded as Dame Winifred Prentice did: 'I feel a bit let down. We thought we were setting up a really first class profession and now they seem to want to throw it away as if we were just factory workers' (Prentice, 1988).

In 1926, 60 years previously, the College of Nursing were saying that a strike over pay would be a 'betrayal of trust ... putting professional advantage before the needs of the people they serve' (Abel-Smith, 1960). This ambivalence about professional or worker status thus lives on.

The General Secretary of the RCN has expressed belief that its members want an alternative to the traditions of blue-collar industrial action. Membership of the RCN has grown by 80 000 since the late 1970s, and is now the largest and the fastest growing nurses' union in the world. The General Secretary was instrumental in the creation of the pay review body for nurses' pay in 1983, and the decision not to strike in 1982, a commitment to rule 12 of the College's no-strike clause. However, the underlying militancy of some RCN members was evident in demonstrations at London teaching hospitals (*Independent*, 6.2.88).

The divisions within the nursing profession are reflected in membership patterns of the unions. Membership of COHSE, NALGO and NUPE comprises mostly junior grade nurses or those from mental handicap or psychiatric hospitals, which have more male staff. Membership of the RCN has a higher representation of senior nurses, and those who are generalists (Bellaby & Oribor, 1980).

The different unions reflect the clash of interests within nursing, between the ranks of junior and senior nurses and managers and between the different branches of the profession (Salvage, 1985). Such diversity creates difficulty in developing common goals for a workforce to give it leadership and professional support (White, 1984).

Senior managers or clinicians?

It was these kinds of tensions that lead many to the view that the best way forward was to develop the clinical aspects of nursing. They believed that the Salmon structures had over-emphasised the managerial element in senior posts, and the perception that the only way to the top was through management. This had tended to distance ordinary nurses from senior nurses who had become 'the bosses', who were separated from clinical practice. The Price–Waterhouse survey (1988) reflected this tendency. While the large workforce had to be managed there was also a pressure to create a distinct group of senior clinicians to give specialist professional support, on the lines of the American Nurse Consultant. A very similar debate had taken place in social work, which had also been subjected to a 'Salmon type' reorganisation at much the same time.

Thus when District and Unit General Managers came to restructure the management arrangements, in the acute hospitals in particular, they became involved in a longer-term debate within nursing itself about the relevance of senior clinical grades. This debate was also about the appropriate level of delegation of responsibility to the Ward Sister (Kinston, 1987; Carpenter, 1977). It was not merely an argument between general managers and nurses but one that nursing was having with itself (Briggs, 1972).

In many ways the issues were modified in the community services. By their nature they are less hierarchical and less like a complex industrial organisation. They are smaller in scale and the individual practitioner has more freedom of action within the organisation.

The gender issue

Another ancestral dispute concerns the vision of nursing as embodying 'female' qualities (Whittaker & Olsen, 1978; Delamothe, 1988).

The evidence suggests that this is a stereotypical view. It is important to remember that the nurse has always worked closely with the doctors, and has, therefore, become gradually more orientated to the medical model of care.

Nurses' relationships with doctors are to some extent conditioned by the sexual division of labour, which in the past was basically a nurse/female and doctor/male dyad. The development of this pattern was a reflection of Victorian social values that upheld patriarchal control of the family. The family relationships between men and women were transferred into the health care environment. Women were 'mothers' and, by the same token, 'carers'. There is almost a biological determinism in the assumptions that lie behind these stereotypes. The analogy then includes doctors as fathers, and patients as dependent children. The doctor/nurse/patient triad therefore represents the family (Game & Pringle, 1983; Garmarnikow, 1978).

As an outcome of this idea, the occupation of nurse was identified predominently as a 'female' one, and idealised in terms of what constitutes a 'good woman' (Delamothe, 1988). Inevitably, idealisation leads to failure. In reality the projected images of nurses are diverse. Most commonly they fall into three stereotypes of handmaiden, battle-axe, and whore (Muff, 1982; Salvage, 1985). These images are reinforced by popular novels or films, with characters such as the sex symbol army nurse, 'Hot-lips' in *MASH*, and the authoritarian punishing senior nurse in *One Flew Over the Cuckoo's Nest*. The *Carry On* films about hospitals ridicule the nurses who fit these stereotypes (Salvage, 1985).

Some writers go so far as to say that in no other workplace are power relations so 'highly sexualised' as they are in hospitals, and that bureaucratic domination is directly reinforced by sexual power structures. The nurse manager who stops wearing a uniform and dons a smart suit becomes identified with managers, and masculine images of organisational control. This is known in women's magazines as 'power dressing'. Although 75 per cent of the NHS workforce is female, 91 per cent of general manager posts are occupied by men (Chiplin & Sloane, 1982). In nurse management, 43–50 per cent of senior posts are occupied by men although they constitute less than 10 per cent of the workforce and only 3 per cent in the inner London teaching districts (Davies & Rosser, 1986). The RCN council membership also reflects this male dominance.

It has been argued that the domination of nursing by men has replaced the old domination by women of a higher class, the matrons (Salvage, 1985). It is difficult to know if this is a male takeover or a female give-away (Nuttall, 1987). The DHSS report suggests that the higher social status of men, derived from outside the organisation, affects the dynamics of the operations within, and is a contributing factor when considering the clustering of men within the leadership ranks of nursing. Davies and Rosser (1986) write that, 'they were being treated as men first and nurses second'.

The predominance of men in psychiatric nursing originally resulted from the need to restrain violent patients before the introduction of psychotropic drugs. However, the female nurses consistently tried to exclude men from their ranks in the past. The hostility to male nurses may have resulted from the feeling that they would threaten the autocratic, bureaucratic structure of nurse discipline, total commitment and low pay, which were valued by the female élite.

The creation of the Salmon structure provided a more friendly environment for ambitious male nurses, because they possessed the characteristics that would enable them to move up the hierarchy more quickly. These were that they were likely to stay longer in the service, work full time, to want to escape low pay, to change their marginal status, and had greater geographical mobility than their female counterparts (Carpenter, 1978).

The Salmon Report was seen by some to be a critique of *female* authority. The new enlarged bureaucratic structures that resulted were more favourable to the spread of trade unionism and weakened the system of patronage that formerly characterised the nursing hierarchy. The upper-class female élite of nursing was quickly transformed in the psychiatric hospitals by male nurse managers of much humbler origins. This resulted in a domination of women by men from *within* nursing, when before, it had been external, mainly from doctors or administrators in managerial roles or positions of authority (Carpenter, 1977).

The recent reorganisation has done little to change the authority structure on the lines of gender differences but, at least, it has now recognised that problems do exist, and strategies to overcome them are being addressed. The setting up of a National Steering Group on equal opportunities for women in the NHS by the Minister of Health in 1986 will perhaps go some way towards creating a better environment for women to move to higher positions (*NHS Management Bulletin*, 1987).

Very few women have been appointed to the most senior NHS management posts (King's Fund College, 1985). Over half the graduates taken on the NHS training scheme were female, but they were three times more likely to leave the NHS after completing a course, and this was usually the result of domestic circumstances. Much the same can be said of medicine where career breaks are also damaging. Part-time workers move less quickly through the system (Mercer, 1975).

The RCN General Secretary was pessimistic about nurses' roles in the top management of the NHS. 'The entire profession renews itself in ten years', and this meant that, 'management was pouring valuable resources down the drain' (Bealing, 1986). As in other organisations, many of the lower-grade management jobs are filled by women. They constitute 44 per cent of the workforce and 20 per cent of managers, but only 2 per cent become company directors (Tongue, 1986).

In summary, gender is a major issue in the organisation of the NHS. It is also an important factor when considering power relationships between occupational groups such as nurses, doctors and managers, and in the analysis of the power bases within professions. The reluctance many nurses felt in applying for general management jobs was associated with the male stereotype of the job and the implications of a 'macho-type' image, or of the cold calculator removed from the caring feminine role. Some of the doubts expressed by general managers about nurses' capacity to manage could be associated with nursing's female image.

In brief: a creative tension?

From one perspective, the tensions made life more difficult for general managers and senior nursing staff who were trying to work out a new kind of relationship. In other ways, the tensions were fruitful. The climate was right for some fundamental changes to occur and general management actually provided a catalyst to seek a way to resolve some of these long-standing dilemmas. The financial crisis meant that there was a strong incentive to reduce the scale of middle management in nursing. Griffiths provided nurses with the opportunity to rethink and renegotiate some of the past divisions of labour. It provided scope for advancement for able young women nurses that they would not otherwise have had. In the succeeding chapters, we describe the process and the outcome in the districts we studied – it is an unfinished story.

In 1859, Florence Nightingale wrote:

> People's expectancies are highly wrought. . . . They think some great thing will be accomplished in six months, although experience shows that it is essentially the labour of centuries – they will be disappointed to see no apparent change, and at the end of twelve months will feel as flat about it as people do on a wedding day at 3 o'clock when breakfast is over.

The struggles of the nursing profession are today inextricably interrelated to the struggles of the NHS as a total organisation. The NHS is trying to respond to profound financial, technological and social pressures in an unstable environment in a short space of time. The capacity for the two organisations to change to meet each other's needs is limited by the constraints each suffers.

4
Professions in the NHS: new perspectives

———————— ◆ ————————

Throughout this study two themes recur. The first is the relationship between a large formal organisation, the NHS, with the professionals such as nurses who deliver the service. The second theme is a debate about structure of management itself, and especially how the different levels of work should be organised. These two themes interact. There is an extensive literature on the sociology of organisations and management theory that addresses these themes, although there are some major deficiencies. In this chapter, some of this work is briefly reviewed to provide a framework for the study findings.

The professions have always posed problems for managers and organisational theorists alike. Similarly, professionals have always had difficulty with formal organisations despite the fact that many of them, including nurses, now work for bureaucratic organisations of one kind or another. Classical writers on management ignored the professions, and early writers on the sociology of the professions either ignored bureaucratic organisations or saw them as alien to the professional ideal. The education and socialisation of the two groups has therefore tended to reinforce the problems of co-existence.

The classical model

Max Weber (1947) described the classical system of bureaucratic control (Bendix, 1971). There were four principal characteristics, namely hierarchy, continuity, impersonality, and the rule of experts. In this ideal type of model, hierarchy was based on the division of

43

labour, each level being accountable to the one above. This pattern created a career structure, and to a large extent, job security. Prescribed rules needed a system that functioned, in theory, without partiality, and experts or professionals were trained to carry out their functions (Bendix, 1977).

Weber's model was one of rationality and was based on the belief that it produced technical efficiency. Its critics have said that rules can become inflexible, impersonality can become indifference, and hierarchy can discourage individuals developing responsibility and initiative. They suggest that Weber failed to realise the ambivalent nature of bureaucracy (Beatham, 1987).

Other writers have suggested that a more organic model was more appropriate. They drew attention to the informal networks of relationships between workers in organisations, and the element of individual participation (Blau, 1972). In order for an organisation to change, it needs an organic structure – a fluid distribution of functions, wide scope for individual initiative and expertise. Attachment to the goals of the organisation should be disseminated rather than concentrated at the top, with individual commitment to professional norms and communication (Beatham, 1987; Burns & Stalker, 1961). These hold good for public as well as private organisations.

The problem about public bureaucracies is that there is no pressure from the market to change their ways to increase efficiency. They are usually monopolistic, so consumers have difficulty in taking their business elsewhere. In the absence of external sanctions, therefore, such bureaucracies can become self-serving because power is vested in individual control of resources, rather than the outcomes (Drucker, 1979).

The biggest problem in public services such as the NHS is the difficulty of actually measuring efficiency and outcomes. For example, qualitative indices of outputs will more often measure efforts to cure rather than measure prevention strategies, which are more problematic to define and assess.

Nevertheless, bureaucracies have their own cultures that embody elaborate codes governing the behaviour of those within, and they incorporate shared assumptions about the aims of the organisation (Peters & Waterman, 1982). But public bureaucracies sometimes perceive themselves as the guardians of national interest and transcending policies of particular governments, and therefore become difficult to change. The problem, as Weber described it, is that bureaucracy can become an 'iron cage' that could prevent innovation, change or risk-taking (Beatham, 1987). General managers were charged with the task of making the NHS an organisation responsive to consumers' changing needs and to the Government demand for efficiency.

The role of the expert or professional

Within bureaucracies or public service systems, the expert or professional has gained power and status. Within health care systems generally, the range of occupations is wide and each is ordered hierarchically (Scott, 1983). The concept of being a professional has certain features. Those most frequently mentioned are that professions have skills based on theoretical knowledge, provision of training, tests of competence, an organisation, a code of conduct, and an ethic of altruistic service.

The emphasis on expert knowledge enables professionals to have freedom and autonomy in their work but this creates problems in an organisation. Etzioni (1969) saw a potential conflict between the structural and sanctioned values of the organisation and the separate internalised 'core values' of professionals that are developed during their training (Atkinson, 1983). Professional high status and disinterested dedication to some extent legitimise the protection from competition in the labour market that they seek. They have a special voice in determining what constitutes a problem in need of expert intervention, for example, doctors influence conceptions of illness (Reuschemeyer, 1983). Nevertheless, this authority of 'special expertise' constitutes a problem for bureaucracy. The experts develop loyalty to their own group, and these may not be the same as those of the career bureaucrat whose loyalty is tied to the organisation itself (Davies, 1983). Public administrative systems stress centralisation of decision-making and formalisation, but professionals stress decentralisation and personal autonomy. Scott (1983) suggests that the conflict lies between administrators in health care systems and planners emphasising macro-criteria, and practitioners/professionals stressing micro-criteria.

The view that professions have of themselves has been strongly influenced by the model created by the medical profession

(Carr-Saunders & Wilson, 1933). A statutory body registers practitioners who are then licensed to offer a professional service. Individuals can be disciplined or 'struck off' the register for lapses in professional conduct and standards.

The professional's values stress doing the very best for a particular client or patient regardless of cost, whereas the bureaucrat is cost conscious. The professional treats each case on its merits using professional discretion to make judgements. The bureaucrat is bound by rules of equity between users. The professional derives authority from his or her access to a body of knowledge, necessarily closed to the non-professional, and is therefore not open to challenge by those outside the profession. The bureaucrat is a generalist who has to weigh experts' views against one another. The professional sets the appropriate standards of practice and disciplines his or her peers. These may not converge with bureaucratic needs, and managers may see the standards as unrealistically high.

Managers also contest the view that only doctors or nurses can discipline themselves. Historically, as medical knowledge deepened and became more specialised, nursing developed its own body of expertise, the power of the professions generally grew relative to that of the lay administrator. This was not confined to health or even to public services. The professions came to occupy an increasingly powerful position as 'knowledge élites' within the social service sector precisely because they delivered the services (Dunleavy, 1987; Wilding, 1982; Hunter, 1988). Their day-to-day decisions determined the way resources were allocated. The State came to lose control of the services it purported to provide as the caring professions perceived themselves as independent organisations within organisations.

The mirror image of these attitudes is reflected in the classical writings on industrial management. For example, Fayol's (1949) basic principles of management were unambiguous. Management is only concerned with corporate goals. Individual and professional interests must therefore be subordinated to the general interest. The manager must exercise complete authority and strict discipline on all those in the part of the organisation for which he is responsible. There must be unity of command. 'For any actions whatsoever, an employee should receive orders from one superior only.' There is no room in this model for a privileged kind of employee with professional autonomy.

The early organisation theorists, concentrated on the *problems* presented by the growth of bureaucracies and the development within them of powerful professional groups. Modern organisations were efficient partly because they had become the repository of expertise, but that expertise was increasingly becoming specialist or fragmented. Yet the legal authority of the organisation continued to reside with the administrator or in modern parlance, the manager. Bendix (1971) put the dilemma succinctly:

> Ultimately, all professional services involve an element of trust in the skill and wisdom with which the professional makes his judgements, whereas accountability of all administrative actions are subject to scrutiny and criticism by higher authority. It is only somewhat exaggerated to say that the trust implicit in the employment of professionals is at odds with the distrust implicit in the accountability of administrators.
>
> (pp. 147–8)

More recently, economists came to reinforce the conflict model. Friedman (1962) and, later, writers from the public choice school of theorists (Mueller, 1979) have argued that the whole notion of professions as altruistic self-regulating collegiate groups is fiction. Their actions are best understood as the expression of restrictive practices. Individuals band together to monopolise knowledge, to restrict entry to the profession and hence put up the price to be paid for that knowledge. Professions have merely extended that exploitation of consumers in the market place to public bureaucracies. They use their monopoly of specialist knowledge to win battles for resources. The cloak of clinical autonomy is merely a disguise for the exercise of group power politics. The flavour of this set of ideas is to be found in political debate in the mid 1980s, and the more general hostility to the professions.

The consensus model

Other work, both on the sociology of professions and organisations, questioned the validity of these original models. It looked more closely at what actually happens on a day-to-day basis between people in organisations. It examined the way informal structures work as opposed to the formal organisation charts.

What emerged was that professional values are more complex than the original stereotypes suggested. Although their education may not prepare them well for this, professionals in health services can appreciate that the organisation's larger goals reflect their common commitment to the individual patient whom the organisation as a whole is serving (Davies, 1983).

Informal patterns of collaboration between professionals were crucial to the working of health care. From this it was deduced that management by consensus was not only possible but was actually practised. These ideas found their way into the 'Grey Book' prescriptions (DHSS, 1972). Like other theories of their time, they played down the importance of conflict – especially in a period of tightening resources and 'zero sum games' when advances by one profession had to be won at the expense of another.

There are also other conflicts between different sectors of the Health Service between geographical interests, between units, between district and region. The consensus model also ignored these conflicts, and others that existed within professions. Professions, early theory predicated, reproduced themselves through a process of socialisation. During this 'training period' core values are internalised. It may be viewed as almost a 'doctrinal conversion' (Hughes, 1958), but this view is now considered to be overstated. It implies an idea of the student as an empty vessel, which is quite false or, at least, oversimplified (Atkinson, 1983).

Studies of medical students (Becker, 1960) and nurses (Davis, 1968) show that often there is a serious misalignment between the expectations of students and those of the profession. The separating of education and service creates conflicts for the nursing student, and such deep uncertainty that this is the cause of many leaving. The self-concept of the profession as expressed through ideological and pedagogical rationale simply did not, in the past, fit practical experience (Davis, 1968).

Currently, there is high value in individual holistic nursing of patients, which in reality may be difficult to accomplish (Schurr & Turner, 1982). This has been described more recently in a British study of nurses in training and the socialization process (Melia, 1987). Confusion exists because there are so many areas of overlap between the tasks that student nurses perform and those done by unqualified nursing auxiliaries. Close analysis of the idea that professions have clear-cut values, ideals and objectives as a corporate group reveals that the reality is far more untidy and contradictory. Professional boundaries often overlap with other groups, particularly in nursing.

There have been other critics of the functionalist interpretations of professional versus organisational values (Dingwall & Lewis, 1983). An examination of nurses' relationships with the health care system and patients illustrates that they may hold professional, bureaucratic and humanitarian ideals all at the same time (Rosenthal, 1980).

Leininger (1970) suggested that nursing was moving from a traditional to a new modern culture. For example, the collective bargaining over pay and conditions for nurses can be interpreted as a rejection of the self-sacrificing norms of the past in the nursing profession. These changing norms bear a relationship to the 'ancestor' role models we discussed in Chapter 3. Ancestor myths, and values incorporated in myths, change and adapt to new external social forces (Douglas, 1987). Delamothe (1988) drew up a list of attitudes of doctors and nurses in terms of binary oppositions (Fig. 4.1).

However, the changing semantics in the debates about the role of nursing in health care systems actually look and sound different to this typology. There has been a shift from the traditional model defined in Delamothe's classificatory system towards new definitions of nursing, which also reflect more closely the norms of the total

Nurse	Doctor
Female	Male
Dependence	Autonomy
Care	Cure
Intuition	Science
Sympathy	Rationality
Low status	High status
'Low-tech'	'High-tech'
Training	Education
Occupation	Profession

Figure 4.1 *Stereotypical attitudes to nurses and doctors*

Past Family Model	Present Bureaucratic Model
Paternalism	Managerialism
Authority	Democracy/equality
Medicalisation	Individual self-help
Task orientation	Holistic approach
Simple technology	Complex technology
Vocation	Professionalism
Undifferentiated workforce	Division of labour
Low status	High status
Obedience	Self-reliance
Dependence	Autonomy
Handmaiden	Industrial worker
Submissive/feminine	Dominant/masculine
Art	Science
Powerless	Powerful
Training	Education
Passive	Active

Figure 4.2   *Key words from texts on nursing*

health care organisation. The words in Figure 4.2 represent binary oppositions between past and present conceptions of nursing. A rough content analysis of recent and past texts on nursing shows that a different pattern of words is being used. Nursing has responded to the changing nature of the Health Service of which it is a part.

The traditional model outlined in discussions about the past is rapidly moving towards the bureaucratic mode, and all the connotations that implies. Modern nursing texts use the language of the bureaucratic model. The semantics used about modern nursing suggest that there is a shift towards a more masculine, bureaucratically defined model of nursing. However, traditional conceptions of the nurse's role still persist in the minds of nurses, and of other groups of NHS employees and the public at large.

The power of those old images was inherent in the RCN anti-Griffiths publicity campaign. The polar opposition they represented is less relevant to the new images of nursing whose value system is converging more closely to that of the organisations in which they work. The problem is that the caring and humanitarian character of nursing in the past also needs to be sustained and incorporated into the image of nursing today.

A new way forward?

If there are divergent and conflicting interests within the Health Service, as well as shared values, what kind of leadership would help promote the shared values and hold a fair balance between the conflicting interests, so that the Health Service serves the interests of the consumer and not the professions? This was the difficult question general managers had to try to answer. They were drawing implicitly and explicitly on new theoretical orthodoxies about how organisations work.

In his classic text on management, Drucker (1979) argued that the essence of the management problem in the non-market service sector was that service managers tended to measure their success not in terms of the quality of the service they provided but by the size of the budget they could command. The essential change that had to be achieved was to turn the organisation at every level into one that was maximising its performance and the quality of the service it provided to its consumers.

Separate professional or functional hierarchies naturally tend to see the world from their own profession's view point and to make this corporate effort difficult. The greater the distance between the front-line professional and the people at the top of the hierarchy, the more this will be the case. Those in the front line working with other professions have the greatest incentives to collaborate. They gain personal satisfaction when team work produces results. The more that responsibility is delegated downwards, the greater the incentives to team work. At the same time, the centre has to be able to hold these individuals to account for their performance, otherwise delegation becomes anarchy.

This can be achieved by delegating financial responsibility, or budget-holding, downwards in return for holding those responsible to account and measuring their performance. The centre must give clear leadership on where the organisation is going and what the overall objectives and values are, holding each sub-unit to account for its contribution to the whole while at the same time making lines of responsibility simple and clear. This is a 'tight and loose structure' in the words of Peters and Waterman (1982). Collaboration and consensus emerges in the small teams or groups who actually deliver the care. This is a move away from the structural functionalist models of organisations of the past towards a more organic approach. Several general managers and nurses, we observed, were working towards the newer conception of management.

Levels of work

A close and extensive analysis of many organisations (Table 4.1), both industrial and social service in character, suggested to one group of researchers that it was possible to discern broad levels of work common to many organisational settings (Jacques, 1978; Billis, 1984; Billis & Rowbottom, 1987; Kinston 1987). At one end of the

Table 4.1   *Levels of work*

Level	Title	Expected work
5	Field coverage	Covering a general field of need throughout a society.
4	Comprehensive provision	Providing a complete range of products or services throughout a whole territorial or organisational society.
3	Systematic provision	Making systematic provision according to the needs of a flow of open-ended situations.
2	Situational response	Carrying out concrete tasks whose precise objectives have to be judged according to each situation encountered.
1	Prescribed output	Carrying out concrete tasks whose objectives are completely specifiable beforehand so far as is significant.

Source: Billis & Rowbottom (1987).

spectrum there are *level one* tasks. These can be reasonably clearly defined in advance and are regular and straightforward. They may involve personal interaction, but not individual professional judgements and discretion. Next there is *level two* work that entails 'situational response' judgements about each individual client or patient's needs, using professional skills.

Part of the dilemma of nursing is that some nursing tasks span both levels one and two. Furthermore, nurses have to work as a team and in collaboration with other teams of nurses as well as other professionals. The teams have different logics depending on the nature of the medical technology or the community setting. The ward is only one obvious organisational setting, an operating theatre another, an intensive care unit another. In these situations the team needs a leader. Whether that leader should be one person for a 24-hour period, (Kinston, 1987) or whether the responsibilities should be shared as the unions argued after the grading restructuring exercise, was a contentious issue. Moreover, a Ward Sister can lead a team of nurses and also be a line manager of other workers in level one jobs such as cleaners.

The next level of work, *level three*, involves analysing the work undertaken at the level below, making sure enough people are in post for the changing demands put on them, assessing priorities and ensuring they are adopted, identifying recurring problems and suggesting solutions. 'The essential job is to develop a systematic response to the flow of changing needs. It means not only dealing with the needs of today but constantly developing the system by which the needs of tomorrow are to be met.' (Billis & Rowbottom, 1987). It is defining and clarifying this level of work that often causes the most difficulty.

Some problems cannot be solved at this level and may require the whole unit to rethink its objectives or priorities on a multiprofessional basis. That is *level four* work – strategic and medium-term over several years. Considering priorities between units, district-wide policies and professional practices and recruitment and training is a *level five* function fundamental and long-term in its implications. Ideally, the theory suggests at each level one person should be responsible for that level of work within a defined organisational boundary such as a hospital, a ward, or community unit.

In practice, this poses practical difficulties and it leaves open for discussion just how to define the range of work to be included.

Should the 'ward leader' lead not just nursing staff but other staff too? Should the service manager be a professional or generalist? How should responsibilities at each level be divided between the dominant professions such as nursing and medicine, and new general managers? Such theories produced no conclusive guidance and general managers had to work out their own solutions.

Griffiths proposals and nursing organisation

In the old management philosophy, organisational authority tended to be seen as the single right to give instructions. Hence no one should serve two masters – unity of command was all. This was implicit in the old Salmon structure and in some versions of general management.

While such 'dual influence' situations are to be avoided whenever possible, they cannot be denied or excluded altogether (Billis & Rowbottom, 1987). Where they do exist it is important to recognise it. For managers and nurses alike, this was a hard lesson that they learned over the period of our study. The loss of the Salmon structure meant that nurses could be responsible to a non-nurse line manager, but that left open their distinct legal and ethical responsibilities as professionals. This problem can be resolved but it is important to recognise the distinct need for a separate source of professional advice and support for nurses whose line manager is not a nurse.

Within the NHS organisation, an independent hierarchy had developed in accordance with the recommendations of the Salmon Report. The main feature of this nursing structure was that the management of nursing was along the lines of professional accountability (see Fig. 1.1). In this system, professional and managerial accountability were seen to be inseparable. The reasons were complex but this was mainly because of the need to square up the accountability of the nurse as an NHS employee, and that of the nurse as an independent professional. The problem lay with the very nature of the nursing tasks.

The very intimate and daily contact with the public that nurses serve gives them an understanding of patients' needs, which is immediately and subjectively experienced. This front-line worker role gives them, like their medical colleagues, personal as well as corporate responsibility for what they do 'to' and 'for' the public. As workers at the interface of the organisation they are especially vulnerable.

Each group of nurses is governed by specific legislation; for example, the Mental Health Acts, the law governing midwifery supervision, the licensing of nursing agencies, laws relating to child abuse, are significant for nurses in different parts of the Health Service. Other legislation that affects the general population has a heightened meaning for nurses who work in settings where a high degree of skill, discipline and accuracy is called for. Personal responsibilities often involve major issues of life and death. The common law of 'personal responsibility', 'vicarious liability' and 'tort', has a special meaning for nurses who often work in environments fraught with the possibility of accidents and mistakes, resulting in serious damage to persons or loss of life (Young, 1981).

For example, the Misuse of Drugs Act 1971 and the 1978 Amendment Order, places particular stress on the role of nurses administering drugs. The 1981 Education Act requires yearly statements from School Nurses and Health Visitors about children with 'special needs'. The 1969 Children and Young Persons Act, and related amendments, places onerous responsibilities on midwives and Health Visitors to identify and care for children defined as being 'at risk'.

Ethical issues are also involved in the process and activity of nursing (Benjamin & Curtis, 1981). The Abortion Act 1967 and the Human Tissues Act 1961 relating to transplanted organs, involve nurses in human problems that are not common to other occupational groups in the NHS, with the exception of doctors. What is more, they are immediate problems that involve the nurse in on-the-spot decision-making, and call for a high degree of personal responsibility at every level.

For these reasons, nurses argued in the past that they needed to be accountable to managers who had an understanding of the issues involved, and needed support from their professional organisations. The issue of managerial accountability is therefore multifaceted. Nevertheless, the concept of general management challenges the logic of professional independence within the NHS and suggests that, above a certain level, there is no necessity for professional line or functional management. This is to encourage a more integrated and organic approach to health care provision. But the issues that are specifically related to professionalism still remain. The creation of an advisory framework for nurse professionals was seen as a strategy for overcoming this structural problem. However nurses challenged the legitimacy of appointing managers without expert knowledge.

The fieldwork analysis in the second part of this study addresses those problems of professional specialism, individual responsibility and the role of advice within the post-Griffiths NHS organisation. The study focuses on one region, and the strategies of nurses and general managers to resolve conflicting conceptions of organisational structure.

PART II
The study

———————— ◆ ————————

Anyone who does not lay his foundations beforehand could do so later only with great skill, although this would be done with inconvenience to the architect and danger to the building.

(Machiavelli: *The Prince*, 1513)

5
Implementing general management

———————— ◆ ————————

Nationally, the principal source of recruitment for general managers was from the administrative sector of the NHS. There were relatively few appointments of doctors, nurses and managers from the private sector (Table 5.1).

Table 5.1   *Former jobs of new general managers in 1986*

NHS general managers	*Regional Health Authorities*	*District Health Authorities*	*Units (hospitals)*
Former NHS administrators	9	132	364
Doctors	1	15	110
Nurses	1	4	70
Outsiders including private sector	3	38	54
Vacancies		2	13
Total	14	191	611

Source: 'National Health Service', *The Economist*, 4.10.86.

Creating a role and its implications for nursing

As we saw in Chapter 1, the expectations placed on general managers were high. Yet the concept of general management as applied to the NHS was rudimentary or non-existent. The Templeton

College Centre for Management Studies at Oxford interviewed a sample of 20 District General Managers over a two-year period as they began their new jobs. They all felt they had to discover for themselves what the job involved. Neither their Chairman nor the DHSS had helped them to do so to any significant extent. The responsibility to achieve change and give direction to the service were key elements for everyone. Templeton (1987) identified several somewhat different perceptions of the role:

- a *monitor* of performance;
- an *initiator* of strategic changes leaving others to carry it through;
- a *symbolic figurehead* setting the tone for the organisation;
- an *organiser*, giving people a sensible organisational framework within which to do their job; and
- a *team leader*, 'the professionalism of most people working in the Service is vital for patient care. If DGMs threaten to bulldoze that, the professionals' morale will fade and therefore so will standards of care. So you must *support* care.'

Who were the District General Managers?

These views found echoes in our own interviews with 14 District General Managers in North West Thames in 1986. Their previous occupations may explain this. Their educational origins were diverse. All but one had a degree, but they varied from engineering and pure science through zoology and geography to economics and social science. One had a diploma in social administration but only four had taken courses in management. Most were aged between 33 and 45 years and had come from within the NHS.

Only four of the fourteen had business backgrounds and all but two were NHS administrators. Of the ten NHS appointments, six were the resident District Administrator, six were products of the National Health Training Scheme and seven had worked primarily in the North Thames Regions. They were experienced in the complexities of the Health Service and were used to working with professional colleagues. None conformed to the stereotype 'businessman with a calculator' image of the RCN public propaganda.

What were their priorities?

The DGMs in our study were each asked to give a list of the major priorities within their districts as they saw them at the beginning of their period in post. At that point, the process of introducing new unit structures was high on their list of immediate tasks – it was 'taken as read'. However, they also listed their fundamental longer-term objectives as summarised in Table 5.2 – some were personal, some were the region's. Most DGMs listed several objectives as their primary concerns. Five mentioned hospital closures and developing priority services as their major task. These objectives had been set before their appointment by their own authorities responding to regional and national guidance.

One insider described his job as, 'delivering the sharp end of regional policy'. An outside DGM had a certain ambivalence about the 'innundations from on high' about policy and objectives and how to deal with them. He felt a personal responsibility to develop his own local objectives after a careful appraisal of the scene. Outsiders faced with initiating major financial changes were at a disadvantage in this respect as they were also mastering the complexities of a local organisation and the NHS in general. They were developing new relationships at regional and district level, and at the same time trying to create a personal view and style. Insiders had already had the chance to do one or all of these things.

Table 5.2   *Major policy objectives of DGMs*

Objectives	Number of DGMs ranking objective as important					
	1	2	3	4	5	6
Closure of hospitals					x	
Developing priority services					x	
Expanding acute services				x		
Reducing acute services			x			
Reducing spending		x				
Creating a capital plan		x				
Introducing information systems		x				
Improving existing stock	x					
Funding for research establishment	x					

Table 5.3   *Organizational objectives of DGMs*

Objectives	Number of DGMs ranking objectives as important						
	1	2	3	4	5	6	7
Right grades of staffing							x
Integration of UGMs and DMB							x
Recruitment of nurses					x		
Training managers/staff				x			
Defining own goals				x			
Effectiveness and efficiency			x				
Fusion of two districts			x				
Reviewing roles of District Officers		x					
New roles of DHA members established		x					
Decentralizing budget control	x						

Managers from business backgrounds were more critical of the organisation of the NHS, pointing out its excessive paperwork, inability to be concise and its propensity for lengthy meetings. These characteristics, they contended, differed from their experience in business or industry. Only two DGMs described the new general management role in terms of being 'radical' and 'biting the bullet', or being 'macho' – and these were both insiders. DGMs were then asked to say what they saw as their more immediate organisational objectives (Table 5.3)

It can be seen from this table that the proper grading of staff including nurses was high on the agenda for nearly half the DGMs. This was two years before the 1988 row about regrading. One manager remarked that the terms of the Whitley Council agreements placed major constraints on attracting high calibre people in a region where experienced managers could earn very high salaries in commerce and industry. This was particularly true of accountants and financial staff.

The need to create a harmonious management team was also strongly articulated. Two DGMs expressed anxiety that units could become self-absorbed and unsympathetic to each others' needs and others forecast difficulties in their relationships with the powerful Unit General Managers. The recruitment of nurses was articulated as a major problem for five of the DGMs. Again, note that this was early in 1986. They stressed the importance of heightening the image of social worth of the nurses. This put priority on attracting new recruits into a service that was heavily deficient. One DGM had created the unusual role of Nurse Advisor and DNE combined. He saw a unity between education, training and maintaining a stable committed workforce. He said his service depended on the success of this key role. We return to this example in Chapter 6.

DGMs differed widely in *what* importance they put on nursing. At the opposite end of the spectrum to the five who gave it top billing, was the alternative view that 'My priorities have nothing to do with nursing here.'

The immediate structural decisions that had to be taken were of three kinds:

● creating a management team at district level;
● deciding on unit structures; and
● appointing Unit General Managers.

These would set the pattern of the Service for years to come and had implications for nursing.

Creating new management structures at district level

This was a necessary first step and District General Managers in this region approached the task in somewhat different ways, reflecting their varied management styles, previous experience of the service and their personal relationships with past colleagues still in post. Broadly, three models of district level management emerged (see Fig. 5.1).

1 *Model 1*: the new District Management Boards were essentially the same bodies as the old consensus district management teams, which included a Chief Nursing Officer or equivalent. All members had executive power.
2 *Model 2*: the directors of Personnel, Planning, and so on normally met with the UGMs and the professional advisors, including the

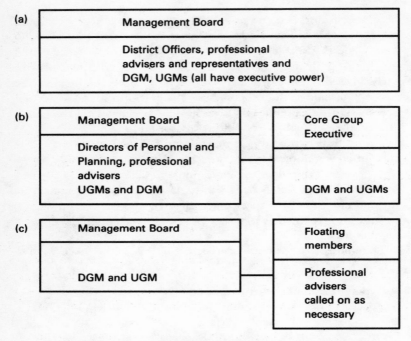

Figure 5.1   *Examples of new management arrangements in North West Thames: (a) Model 1; (b) Model 2; and (c) Model 3*

nurse. But a core group of general managers held the executive power and met as a core group.

3   *Model 3*: was the most altered. The core group, the DGM and the Unit General Managers, met regularly and only called others in as necessary. Here the Management Board consisted only of general managers. This model was short-lived.

As these examples show, the new post of District Nurse Adviser (DNA) could occupy a central role or an ambiguous or peripheral one. Precisely how these roles worked out in practice is discussed in Chapter 6.

Creating new unit structures

Once the new district management structures were in place, each district had to be subdivided into units of management. This could

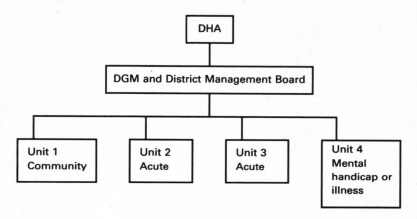

Figure 5.2   *A typical district structure*

mean, for example, that the district general hospital became one unit, a long-stay hospital another and the community services a third (Fig. 5.2) As one DGM put it, the primary objective of the reorganisation was to delegate operational responsibility to the unit:

> The units will not be given the options of referring these matters for resolution by the district-based management board. . . . District level functions exist only as long as they can demonstrate their practical capacity to provide assistance to UGMs.
>
> (Best, 1985)

This was a clear expression of the philosophy underpinning the Griffiths proposals. Units were to be the key focus for operational management, 'getting things done'.

Unit General Managers

Nationally, the new group of Unit General Managers, nearly 700 of them in 1987, had come predominantly from administrative backgrounds (Disken *et al.*, 1987), and 82 per cent were men. Over half came from the same health authority. Men were even more heavily represented in the acute units where nearly 90 per cent were male.

Table 5.4   *The Backgrounds of UGMs in NWT in 1985–6*

District or Regional Administrative Officers	23		
Consultants/Community Physicians	3		
Nurses	8	Inside district	20
External recruits	5	Outside district	17
Pharmacists	1	Unknown district	3
Total	40		

Most UGMs we interviewed in North West Thames came from inside the NHS (Table 5.4). We asked why more nurses were not appointed. Most DGMs said that it was because very few actually applied for the UGM posts, and cross checking with the data on applicants showed this to be true. Most applications were from administrators or industrial managers. Sometimes, nurses were approached and invited to apply for these posts, but were reluctant to compete. Nurses were said to fare less well in the selection process because their training was considered too narrow.

One DGM said that in shortlisting UGMs, it was necessary to 'play the game' and have the 'token nurse, administrator, and so on' in order to make the process balanced and fair. However, in many instances DGMs had already identified a candidate personally, although the selection committee made the ultimate decision. Only one DGM complained that his choice on a particular occasion was overriden by the selection panel.

In some cases, the field was very limited and the DGM felt that the best must be made of local talent. In situations where a second round of interviewing was necessary in order to fill a UGM post, the DGM had usually first identified someone personally, and invited him or her to apply. This was the case for at least six UGMs.

Most DGMs said that paper qualifications, as such, were not an important basis for selection. Track record of proven good management was the main criteria, and professional background secondary. Personal qualities ranked highly and were pithily conceptualised in terms of 'a fixer', 'an analytical thinker', 'a conciliator', 'a decision maker'. Most DGMs stressed they had attempted to fit the personal qualities of a UGM to the needs of the structure.

The 'outsider' DGMs were no more or less likely than their NHS colleagues to appoint an outsider like themselves. One DGM in this category, however, stressed that he felt a real need to have 'insiders' because of his own lack of health experience. Alternatively, an insider DGM said it was important to have at least one outsider UGM to 'ask the unaskable, to think the unthinkable'.

Variability in new unit structures

No specific format was suggested in the Griffiths proposals for organisational structures. Directions for change were implicit rather than explicit. Managers should be appointed regardless of discipline, and greater freedom given to organise according to local requirements. The further away from direct patient care, the less important it became to have skills related to professional disciplines. The nearer management gets to the patient the more important it is for the doctors to be 'the natural managers' (Griffiths, 1983). These statements left in doubt as to what level above the ward general management should begin, and what role should be allocated to nurse managers. The Service was moving from a 'role' orientated philosophy to a 'task' orientated one.

Once Unit General Managers (UGMs) were appointed, they, in turn, had to decide how to structure their units – how far to extend the principle of general management, and whether to keep the separate nursing management hierarchies that had existed. Should they appoint a Director of Nursing Services for the hospital or not?

Some UGMs concluded that, to a larger extent, nursing services within acute units could be left much as they were. Others decided that the principle of general management ought logically to be extended right through the system and that there should be *no* senior nurses managing nurses above ward level. A hospital could be divided into sub-units, just as a district could be divided into units and one person, a sub-unit or Service Manager to be given clear control of everything that happened there. One division of activity might be inpatient services, another might be outpatient, accident and emergency, another laboratory or support services.

Many unit managers responsible for community services also felt that the Griffiths logic suggested that their services could best be organised on a 'locational' not a professional or occupational basis. A new UGM often meant a restructured service. Once again, senior- and middle-management nurses were caught up at the heart of these changes. It is a mistake to believe, as some outsiders do, that general management stopped with the appointment of DGMs and UGMs, and that 'it all happened in 1986'. In many areas, the structural changes went on well into 1987 and, in some units, structures and responsibilities were unresolved even in 1988. There had been three years of uncertainty and change.

General management establishes itself

General managers we spoke to in 1986 knew that a great deal was expected of them and were only too aware that they were caught in the middle of powerful countervailing forces, central government policies, regional imperatives, local pressures. They had to prove themselves quickly. They were on short-term contracts of three or four years mostly. Their performance was to be judged and graded by their District Chairman and the Regional Chairmen. Although they stressed the long-term nature of the changes that had to be made, creating the units and choosing the staff had taken 12–18 months – nearly half their first contract period. One DGM commented that short-term contracts led to:

> playing safe, and not really solving the problem of getting rid of people, or taking a risk for fear of offending people. The role of the DGM is difficult to define to the DHA, it involves so much exertion of pressure on other people, and engenders so much anxiety and uncertainty . . . I am the only one to have some degree of control over myself.

For those DGMs who were formerly the resident DA, matters of existing personal DMT relationships posed further problems:

> They were my friends, now my role is different. Before we were equals, now it is unequal. Now I am personally responsible for poor managers, therefore I must push the ineffective person out, and that is difficult, but my own performance depends on their expertise and effectiveness.

Nearly all DGMs identified the key relationships to be with the Chairman of the DHA. In addition, there was a powerful link with the Regional General Manager (RGM). For most DGMs there seemed to be considerable uncertainty as to what criteria, if any, would eventually be used to assess their performance. One DGM said that the region acted as 'broker', taking money from one district and locating it in another. However, if this proved politically embarrassing, it might backtrack. In these circumstances, a DGM could be seen to fail in the eyes of his DHA for no fault of his own. These views were close to those reported in the Templeton Study (1987).

In his reflections to the introduction of general management, the distinguished American observer of the Health Service, Alan Enthoven, was sceptical that anything would be fundamentally changed: 'There is a real danger they will be little more than cosmetic ... the distinction between general manager and team approaches is a matter of shades of grey. There is less than meets the eye.' (Enthoven, 1985).

Certainly, they were constrained by external pressures as Victor Paige the first Chairman of the National Supervisory Board had experienced. Early interviews reflected areas of potential conflict and were reminiscent of the parallel that Gluckmann (1970), the anthropologist, drew between the Zulu warrior hierarchy and modern industrial enterprise. The Zulu chiefs stood between colonial rule and their own people. The DGM stands between region and district. Managers experience 'unresolved authority conflict' and suffer from 'a frailty of authority', in other words, trying to please those above and below sometimes in contradictory circumstances. Power lies with national politicians, with consultants and with the trade unions and the local DHAs. They have to legitimise their authority by their own efforts.

Yet, at the end of our study when re-interviewing DGMs, we found that most had come through their first testing period and had become accepted. General management had begun to give the Health Service direction despite the very difficult financial climate. This was the RGM's view:

> There is no doubt that the introduction of general management into the NHS has become a significant success story. There has been a profound management change. In the past, a good manager in the NHS was judged by success with processing of the organization; now, he or she is judged on results. The change has enabled a massive release of managerial energy. We

now have a more efficient management system at local level,
which is increasingly achieving better value for money and
providing opportunities to develop a more entrepreneurial
spirit.

According to David Kenny at the King's Fund International
Seminar in June 1988: 'It is unlikely that the financial pressure
could have been withheld without the general management system
in place.' An experienced observer also saw the achievements as
major and unforeseen:

> What I have concluded . . . is that whatever else may be true
> about the introduction of general management, its impact on
> the service has been *immense*. In just five years, an organisation
> that employs more people than any other (non-military) public
> sector organisation in the world . . . has been transformed from a
> classic example of an administered public sector bureaucracy
> into one that increasingly is exhibiting the qualities that reflect
> positive purposeful management.
>
> (Best, 1987)

Confusing priorities

The DGMs themselves felt that the hierarchical controlling aspects
of NHS organisation needed 'loosening up' as too much control still
rested at the top, and there was not enough delegation downwards,
thus limiting their capacity to manage. 'We are swamped by
different priorities being manufactured by the DHSS – "a flavour of
the month attitude". In the end you have to sort out a few things
that are achievable.' It was hoped that the NHS Review would give
more independence to districts. One DGM put the problem more
generally:

> What are we to do, do we respond to all these directives quickly
> or cautiously? The minister may crack the whip now, but it is
> very confusing sometimes, as at a government level one lobby
> will defeat another, the minister changes and you end up feeling
> perplexed.

Talking about the future, the DGMs were also cautious:

There'll be two more reorganisations before I'm through, what's the point in planning or worrying? The format keeps changing, this has the negative effect of giving you the short-term view, it shortens your horizons unfortunately.

There is the ideology now of you've got to keep moving, but that's not good for the NHS. It needs stability as much as change. Too much change at the top is destabilising. New DGMs moving may take their own men, decimating existing managerial staff, leaving a trail of dead bodies, it is not good for the organisation as a whole.

The very personal relationship with DHA Chairmen was another aspect of the new organisation that caused uncertainty about the future. One DGM said: 'You need a sensitively aware Chairman, someone you can get on with.' Another said, 'If you move on, you do not throw up lightly your relationship with your Chairman if it is good.'

The four DGMs in our special review districts were engrossed in the tasks they had set themselves, and would have to be convinced that a DGM post elsewhere would offer the same opportunities to develop their talents. One said 'Where else is there to go that would be better for me?' Yet there was a vague unarticulated expectation that DGMs should move around at least every five years. The uneasy division of power between the districts and the region persisted. One DGM said:

> Really the system is dishonest, as power is emanating from above, and my DHA to some extent is in service to the survival of the district in terms of meeting higher external sanctions. It would be better if there was an honest acceptance of centralised control that already exists covertly.

DGMs also expressed worries about the performance review procedures, as the criteria used were still ill-defined, and the process shrouded in secrecy. It was hoped that this would become clearer in the future when the procedure was better established.

General managers and nursing

Three years after the appointment of the DGMs, the first interviews were followed up in the four selected districts that had been intensively studied in the second phase of the research project. Each district presented different and individual problems for DGMs to solve, some involving major change and others, while maintaining stability, needed more minor adjustments. The gap between the two sets of interviews was about two-and-a-half years.

The DGMs in each district discussed their present role, and in particular their relationship with nursing as follows:

District A

In this district, the DGM was the the ex-District Administrator. He kept the previous Chief Nursing Officer role and kept that title but with added responsibilities of Director of Quality Assurance and inpatient services manager. This hybrid role and others will be described more fully in the next chapter. The DGM explained his reasoning thus:

> If a good and able person was already within the organisation, then it was important to create a role that would fit that person's abilities and meet the organisation's needs. That had been the case in this district. If no such person existed then I would have structured the post differently. The exciting thing about the post-Griffiths situation was that no role had to be preconceived. It could be invented. That was the general manager's choice up to a point, at least, as there was, on some occasions, considerable interference from region and the RCN.

The large nursing workforce was, on its own, sufficient to justify someone at district level to take overall responsibility. His CNO had provided leadership within nursing and made a very positive contribution to general management. Each unit now had an identifiable head of nursing, and the best people had been chosen from within the Service. This required a nurse in a central position to give advice on appointments.

DGM A had tried to involve doctors in the process of general management. There had been a long delay in appointing Service Managers in the acute hospitals while management tried to persuade clinicians to take on the tasks. However, finally these roles had been filled by nurses. He said:

Doctors are afraid to be 'Clinical Directors' or 'Service Managers' because they are afraid of trying to manage colleagues. They much prefer that others are in charge, then they can use their cave-man tactics to resist the system without upsetting other doctors. I have introduced a new young bright general manager who is tough, they complain but they respect him, and he has managed to make a lot of changes.

DGM A wanted 'the pre-eminence of the Ward Sister' restored. He said that the introduction of information technology was an important step in the process, but it was more important to change attitudes in nursing first. He gave an example of changing the attitude of line managers in the supplies department:

I ask them to go and see the Ward Sisters regularly, ask them if they are receiving a good service, and attend to problems. In the past, supplies was an oligarchy, rather like cleaning, self-sufficient and uncooperative with the people they were meant to be helping like the nurses. Now their attitudes are changing and the service has improved tremendously.

District A has four large mental-handicap and psychiatric institutions within its boundaries, all with serious staffing problems. The movement towards community care required an enormous drive to change attitudes of staff, patients and parents. Recently, a new community home had been set up for children, but problems with nursing staff complements still persisted as there were discrepancies between the pay for Social Service workers in the same field who earned more.

The problem for the DGM was that two policies in the field of mental handicap coexisted. There was the need to upgrade and improve existing facilities at the same time as moving people out into the community, both needing funding. Unfortunately, he said, this was low on the political agenda, and therefore constantly starved of resources.

A recent Telford study in the area revealed that some nurse staffing levels were below minimum requirements. The DGM had undertaken several visits to the hospitals to see for himself. He had come away struck by the 'marvellous job nurses were doing' in view of the pressures they were under, although over the past three years some of these pressures had been eased. There was less overcrowding and patient numbers had been reduced but staff needed to see that longer perspective in order to maintain morale, and that again meant strong leadership. 'There are so many good things that have happened, we really need to communicate these to people,' he said, 'but it's difficult because expectations of the public and the region change every year.'

The Nurses' Grading Review had highlighted many of the anomalies in the funding system:

> Here we need extra money as the large number of long-stay institutions skewed the figures because, in the acute sector, with nursing schools and more learner nurses to help, shortages were less of a problem than in the mental handicap areas with more a severe recruitment and retention crisis.

Nevertheless, overall, he concluded that the Service had improved since the introduction of general management:

> The whole ethos of the NHS before was that you must 'side-foot' and not 'be caught in possession of the ball'. The problem was that it was always someone else's fault if things went wrong, now you appoint people to take responsibility.
>
> As a DGM, I personally feel more commitment and responsibility than I did before. I would like the contractual arrangements to be longer because I want to see some things through. I think that DHAs need that stability and support. But the greater responsibility brings greater pressures, and I certainly feel sometimes that the enjoyment factor has dropped somewhat over the last few years ... there's a lot more aggro ... but it's all very stimulating.

District B

In this district, as in District A, the DGM was the previous District Administrator. He too thought that general management has led to quicker decisions. Whether they were better than before was impossible to say but the atmosphere had changed over the last three years. People had come to accept the DGM in a leadership role.

It is not something that happens overnight. You have to sell it calmly, slowly and with the minimum of upset, then you can change the system. People really *wanted* leadership in the past. I have personally always advocated a Chief Executive role in the NHS, I now feel fulfilled.

The Government had authorised that leadership role but it was no good sending out edicts to consultants. 'You still need consensus, as the consultants still have the capacity to outflank you.' DGMs had to earn their authority.

In this district, the previous CNO had also remained in post but in a new hybrid role with a general management task added on. This DGM had in the first interview not anticipated 'too much revolution here', and that change was going well without too much in the way of authoritarianism. The district was a large one, but most acute problems were in hand at the outset. He felt that a pure advisory role was not enough for his CNO, but wanted to retain her at district level because of her 'competence, willingness and general ability, which fitted into the District Management team'.

He discussed the problems of being an insider DGM, where formerly it had been 'a bunch of equals'. He had felt it difficult to break friendships, but recognised the competing need to gain ascendency over colleagues without causing too much friction. By the second interview, this problem had largely been resolved. He acknowledged that nursing had become an important issue for all health authorities. 'The grading review has put nursing back on the map, and there is now a recognition that attitudes towards nurses must change.' He felt that managers in the NHS had been slow to accept the changing role of women. Modern Ward Sisters, for example, were different from their earlier counterparts – there were limits to what they could accept. 'There is no longer the commitment that existed in the past because more are married and have to divide their time between work and family', he said.

The senior nursing hierarchy who had, in the past, often been unmarried, had failed to recognise or respond to their married colleagues' needs. He felt that the public image of nursing had changed because more men exercised power at the top of the unions adopting a 'street fighter/politician' approach.

The recent conflicts over the grading review and the national guidance that there must be 'one manager in charge' had created resentment. 'It's all to do with the meaning of words,' he said, 'the recommendations can be variously interpreted by the Ministry. The problem is that this has caused a great deal of unhappiness and resentment and nurses feel that management is to blame. The union leaders must bear some responsibility.'

He wanted to introduce ward budgeting, which would enable managers at ward level to arrange staffing themselves. A computerised information system at nursing middle-management level would be a great advance. A daily analysis would help identify gaps and shortages and permit borrowing to be made from other areas. He had seen this in operation in another district. It had worked very well, introducing greater flexibility and personal responsibility:

> You see what happens is that Staff Nurse X wants to take her child to the dentist. Under the present rigid structure of staffing, she will probably take the day off 'sick', but if she is personally sorting it out with her Ward Sister, she will be more likely to arrange to come in later, and they can adjust the work accordingly.

It was evident, comparing this interview with the one over two years earlier, that nursing was higher on the general managers' agenda and that the emphasis was now on devising a management system that would suit the nurses. Moreover, the emphasis had shifted away from the role of the District Nursing Adviser to sorting out staffing problems at the level of the Ward Sister and in middle management and on introducing information systems.

District C

This DHA was a RAWP loser and had a large overspend. This had meant initiating bed reductions and closures among other things. DGM C was an administrator who was appointed from another district. When he took over, the nursing shortages and morale in the district were very acute, and he did not appoint the in-house CNO to the post of DNA. In the first interview, one of his highest priorities was to get nursing right in his DHA. Towards this end, he decided to create a new role and then try to find someone to fill it.

His main concern was with the gap between service and education in nursing. He felt that, by drawing together these two aspects of nursing, he would find some answers to the problems. The need to find a good leader for the nursing service led him to head-hunt for the right person to fill the role he had designed at district level.

In each unit a nursing leader role was also retained, although the Directors of Nursing Services (DNSs) at this level were given hybrid roles with a general management content. At middle-management level, Service Manager posts were created to give a more powerful and attractive image to those jobs. Of the nine senior posts that existed when this DGM took office, eight are occupied by new people.

Removal of some senior nursing staff had taken longer than he had hoped, but personal circumstances had to be taken into account in some cases. The appointment of a DNA/DNE had shown remarkably positive results in this district, and will be discussed more fully in the next chapter. The DGM was satisfied that over the past two years, the status and standing of the district with the English National Board (ENB) had vastly improved. He thought that one of the keys to success had been creating 'significant senior posts' in each unit.

There had been a move to internal shift rotation in two out of three of the local acute hospitals. All new staff were taken on with the understanding that they participate, and existing staff could participate if they wanted to do so. It is a system that the DGM felt had really done a great deal to raise standards. The introduction of information technology (IT) in the acute hospitals, and forward information planning (FIP) in the community services, had done much to improve information systems and the relationship between nursing manpower and patient dependencies.

Over the 3 years, better data on nurse staffing had improved the capacity of management to manage. DGM C said that he felt that the general management structures demanded of people working in the Service an ability to change. New staff were chosen with that in mind. Management had needed to be more sensitive to nurses' needs, creating more opportunities for those at Sister level and creating withdrawal systems for nurses working in more stressful areas of the service.

DGM C said that he thought that the medical staff not the nurses were the least well-equipped to change. Their job security and financing made them very resistant to change: 'I am often surprised when talking to groups of them how unaware they are of each other's clinical practice or specialities. They are very individualistic members of the organisation.'

This DGM had followed through the original high priority he had given to nursing. This was interconnected with his other major concern – that of reducing his authority's overspend. Economies had to be achieved without increasing staff instability and nursing shortages. In the next chapter the strategies used by the DNA in these circumstances will be explored more fully.

District D

This DGM's priority had been set by region, namely 'to deliver the RHA strategy for reducing acute services in inner London'. This was undeniably the hardest job a DGM could be asked to do, as he had to overcome powerful vested interests and hostility. The strategy involved the closure of five hospitals and the development of one.

DGM D had been the District Administrator in one of the districts that formed District D. The two had been merged in 1982, so he was both an insider and an outsider in some respects to the district, and the organisation was still recovering from that fusion. He said that some areas of the district were in 'a shambles' with big overspending that had to be checked. In view of these overwhelming tasks to be accomplished, nursing was low on his list of priorities.

During the following year, the existing CNO left to take up another post, and the district was left without a nurse leader, although an Assistant CNO remained, she had no other role and was left 'floating in organisational space'. A DNS in one of the acute units was appointed to act as the DNA, but for reasons that will be outlined in the next chapter, this was not a satisfactory solution. Ultimately, after a year a new appointment was made, but after a relatively short time the newcomer left; the debate thus ensued as to the best possible way to fill this top post, or whether to fill it at all. Opinion was divided, not least among the nurses.

Ultimately, DGM D said he felt there was a need for a nurse at the district level, and a new role was emerging in view of the major task of commissioning and setting up a new acute hospital in the future. The needs of the district were becoming clear, and it was important to find a nurse with the right skills to fulfil those needs.

DGM D had had a strong CNO in the past, and there had been a good working relationship. The introduction of general management had forced a rethink on this role when the CNO left. He said:

> Before, there was a tendency to have the nurse on the DMT as a comfortable figurehead for the DHA to refer to. In the past, so many were weak and ineffectual people in action, and only a few were outstanding. The education of both nurses and doctors is too narrow in an organisational sense. At the clinical level, they have very little experience or knowledge of the wider organisation. Why then should we expect them to change suddenly into general managers? Outstanding people exist, but here we have a problem. The DHA are thinking in terms of the past conception of the role, I am keen to introduce definite general management involvement in the role, and the unit DNSs refuse to acknowledge that it is necessary or give credibility to the role.

This DGM raised interesting questions about the necessity for, and functions of, a CNO or DNA at district level, and refused to gloss over the ambiguities raised by the post-Griffiths structures in relation to professional hierarchies. These will be examined further in the next chapter.

His major task, to close a large London teaching hospital, and four other smaller hospitals, had moved so far as drawing a plan to put before the Secretary of State. This had taken most of his time and energy. He had explained his strategy to all the major groups of employees within his district, and the logic and thinking behind the exercise. The fact that he had gained a high level of acceptance from professionals and his DHA was a singular and remarkable achievement. Challenging the status quo in nursing was in keeping with a manager who saw himself first and foremost an agent of change, and who had an iconoclastic approach to management. Nevertheless, he too had been forced to give nursing and its management problems a much higher place in his concerns than he expected at the beginning of his period in office.

Nursing moves higher up the agenda

By the end of the first three years in office the DGMs that we re-interviewed were well-versed in the problems of nursing. Those who had been dismissive of the importance of nurse management had been forced by circumstances to take a very different view. They all felt changes were required throughout the structure of nursing that would better meet the needs of ordinary nurses. Most saw this as a much more long-term process than had been first envisaged.

All accepted that nursing needed leadership at various levels. The DGM without a leader of nursing at district level for over a year, had come to the conclusion that a post was necessary. The problem for all DGMs lay in *defining* that new role, and giving it a general management context. There was a tension between high level leadership and centralism and the Griffiths philosophy of devolving line management down to the lowest possible level in the structures. Over the three-year period, the necessity of having a high-level general manager with nursing experience has become more evident, particularly in districts with acute shortage and turnover rates.

General managers recognised the tensions in the Griffiths structures. There was a dual tendency towards centralisation and devolution, a need for professional expertise at a high level but a counter need for the wider view, a need for control to be exercised at the top of the structure and an equal one for empowerment and responsibility to be maintained at the bottom. These tendencies exist in most organisations. They reflect the kind of thinking discussed in the previous chapter – what Peters and Waterman (1982) called the 'loose-tight properties', of a successful enterprise. The focus of attention was therefore shifting to the nature of middle management and support for frontline nursing staff.

Summary

1 Most of the DGM appointments were ex-NHS administrators. The two outsiders who had come from industry had left by the end of the three-year research period. Difficulty of adjusting to the 'culture' of that organisation was greater for outsiders brought in to initiate change.

2 Priorities for local services were set by region and by district, or defined personally by the DGM. The new managers were therefore faced with a complexity of external pressures, which were backed up by financial sanctions. The expectations were that DGMs should meet targets set by region, failure to do so could mean loss of job.

3   In spite of the macho image of managers, the idea of consensus management and team effort was part of the NHS culture, and the new managers sought to achieve their objectives by agreement.

4   Some DGMs put nursing high on the agenda, the majority did not in the early stages of general management. However, over the 3 years, DGMs had become convinced of the importance of good strong, nursing leadership.

5   Some early DMB structures marginalised the role of the professionals in decision-making. The UGMs and DGM in most districts formed a core group who implemented decisions more generally discussed at DMBs. This created a tighter structure, and located power in the hands of a few key people.

6   Appointments of UGMs were not always based on a wide and rational choice.

7   Unit structure changed at different rates, some remained unchanged. Nevertheless, the Griffiths reorganisation left the question of change and models of organisation open-ended. This perpetuated uncertainty, as the changes in 1982 had been quite radical.

8   DGMs who were vested with authority by the region, in reality had it in name only. They had to legitimise that authority by being seen to lead and manage. They were beset by pressures externally from government, region and district, and internally from powerful professional groups.

9   The DGM's key relationship was with the Chairman of the DHA; other important relationships existed too, notably with the RGM. This conflict was particularly apparent in the performance review procedures.

10   General management at the end of three years had become accepted and established. Most DGMs felt that it was an improvement on past organisational forms. However, DGMs felt constrained by a strong tendency to centralism, coupled with a countervailing philosophy of local autonomy. The DGM stood between those polarities, which were inherent in the Griffiths structures.

11   Attempts to involve doctors as general managers had largely failed in the four districts studied. Thus the Griffiths objective was not realised in this respect.

12   Each DGM had introduced his own conception of nurse
     leadership at the district level. There was a considerable
     diversity of views. Most DGMs opted for a hybrid role of CNO
     or DNA coupled with a general management role. One DGM
     questioned the need for such a role at district level. It was clear
     that questioning the status quo in the nursing hierarchy was a
     process that created enormous conflict and pressures to main-
     tain existing systems.

6

An endangered species: nursing advice at district level

———————— ♦ ————————

In Chapter 3 we referred to the past struggles nurses had had to achieve comparable status with the other major status holders in health care, the doctors and the administrators. The post-Salmon changes and nurses' inclusion in the new consensus management teams were an important achievement, even if, in practice, some members were more equal than others.

Given the hierarchical nature of the NHS, any changes to the status of nurses in these senior management roles was only too obvious, and had profound symbolic implications for the profession's image of itself. The early failure to include the Chief Nursing Officer at the DHSS on either the Supervisory or the new NHS Management Board was the first indication that troubles lay ahead. She was later appointed to the former following protests and the House of Commons Report (House of Commons, 1984). Nevertheless, the demotion of one Regional Nursing Officer (RNO) to 'third in line', accountable to a Director of Personnel, was viewed as an explicit attempt to 'downgrade nursing'. (*Nursing Times*, News, 1985).

Under the previous arrangements, a Chief Nursing Officer (CNO) had existed in each District Health Authority (DHA). The Salmon Report (1966), to which we have already referred, had argued that all aspects of professional standard setting, policy formation, advice giving and the managerial control of the workforce were best combined with authority emanating ultimately from a CNO. More specifically, the CNO had six functions:

1   Giving professional advice to the authority on all matters relating to the nursing service and articulating nursing interests,

'the nursing voice', in the determination of the DHA's strategy;

2   Taking responsibility for external relations with professional bodies including cases of professional misconduct, and ensuring compliance with statutory duties imposed on nurses – for example, under the Children's and Young Persons' Acts or the Misuse of Drugs Acts;

3   Maintaining and improving professional standards of practice throughout the Authority's service;

4   Ultimate responsibility for recruitment and training of staff, including nurse education;

5   Management/command and control (including dismissal) of staff; and

6   Functional budget-holding responsibility for nursing.

Yet, as we have seen, the whole thrust of general management was to decentralise day-to-day management functions down to the unit level, giving each Unit General Manager (UGM) the final responsibility for all the staff, service delivery and expenditure of his or her unit (Fig. 6.1). The change is from a rectangular lineal management form in the pre-Griffiths structures to a pyramid-shaped structure in the post-Griffiths organisation.

The Griffiths message was clear: general managers had been asked to:

> Review and reduce the need for functional management
> structures, at all levels from unit management to chief officers at
> Authority level, and ensure that the primary reporting
> relationship of functional managers is to the general manager.
>
> (para. 6)

And it was general managers who were:

> To carry forward the DHSS work, stimulated by the
> management enquiry, in determining optimum nurse
> manpower levels in various types of unit, having regard to the
> needs of the local situation and the maintenance of professional
> standards, so that regional and district Chairmen can
> fundamentally re-examine each unit's nursing levels.
>
> (para. 9.6)

(*a*) Pre-Griffiths Consensus Management Team (DMT)

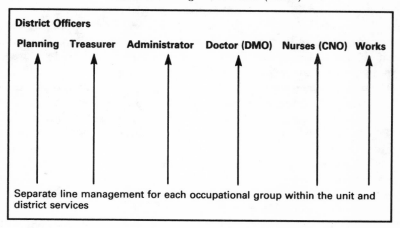

(*b*) Post-Griffiths General Management Structures

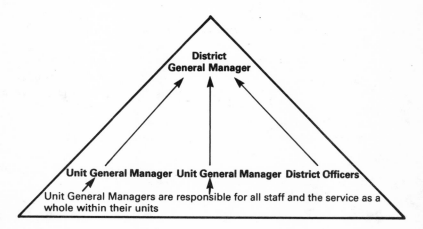

(*a*) is a horizontal shape where decision-making is shared laterally by officers responsible for particular occupational groups.

(*b*) is a pyramid-shaped structure where managers at each level take personal decisions and responsibility for a service and all types of personnel.

Figure 6.1   *Changes   in   a   district   organisation;   (a)   pre-Griffiths: (b)   post-Griffiths.*

For the new general managers, the implications for the post of CNO at district level were therefore critical. They argued that the CNOs functions (5) and (6) above would disappear, becoming the responsibility of the new UGMs. Given the importance attached to the personnel function by Griffiths, function (4) could, it was assumed, be taken over by personnel officers and education left to the nurse educators. Functions (2) and (3) were most appropriately handled by a Director of Nursing Services (DNS) at *unit* level. This left only function (1) – the giving of professional advice to the DHA. It was thought that this was not a time-consuming task and could well be undertaken in combination with another major job. It would, some general managers felt, amount to, at most, one day a week of an individual's time.

These views were not universally held but they summarise a widespread view. Nevertheless, the nursing profession was bringing pressure to bear on politicians nationally. In response to this, the Secretary of State wrote to Trevor Clay, then General Secretary of the RCN, in March 1985 to reassure the College that proper arrangements for nursing advice would be made.

The DHSS subsequently sent 'guidance' to Health Authorities. They were to have 'a single designated source of professional advice at senior level with direct access to the District General Manager and Health Authority itself'. This advice was followed by a letter from the Minister for Health, Barney Hayhoe in November 1985 reiterating that authorities should have 'proper arrangements' for professional advice. While tempted to do away with any nursing responsibilities above the unit they would have to designate someone to be a nursing adviser for the district.

The first round of changes

In the fourteen districts in North West Thames Region, four CNOs were phased out in the first flush of reorganisation. In three districts there was an explicit policy to have no post at all at district level. In these circumstances, the responsibility of giving the nursing advice to the district authority was designated as an additional function for a DNS/DMS working in a local unit or for a nurse who happened to be a UGM. Most of the nurses who remained in district level posts were given other general management responsibilities and

Table 6.1   *DNA roles in North West Thames in 1985–6*

DNA/Director of Quality Assurance	5
DNA/Consumer Relations/CNO	1
DNA/Director of Personnel	1
DNA/Director of Nurse Education	1
DNA/UGM/DQA	1
DNA/DNS	3
DNA/UGM	2
Total	14

undertook nursing advice as an addition (see Table 6.1). The most common arrangement was the combination of DNA with the new and relatively undefined task of 'quality assurance', which we discuss later.

The variety of these dual or hybrid roles reflects the spirit of Griffiths. Each post was fashioned by the DGM to fit the needs of a particular district, or a particular person. As we saw in the previous chapter, the changes in the CNO role also meant a changed relationship with the district management structures. It was no longer a matter of course that the DNA would be an equal and accepted member of the District Management Board (DMB).

In the course of interviews given shortly after the initiation of general management in early 1986, five DGMs said they thought that the role of the DNA at district level would be an anomaly in the future organisation of districts. Some said that the hybrid roles had been invented in their own districts to suit existing CNOs who had proved their worth in the past, and it was felt important to keep them as valuable members of the new teams. Subsequently, three CNOs left for other posts. Those who were thought to have failed, were quickly got rid of, unceremoniously. There was a strong impression among senior nurses that nursing advice, as a district level post, would soon disappear. This impression made recruitment to the remaining posts difficult.

There were, however, some examples of relative stability. The old CNO took on the advisory title with little change in his or her work. This principally occurred in those districts where the existing District Administrator (DA) had been given the post of DGM. Such an arrangement had the advantage of continuity but had the disadvantage of limiting experimentation with new concepts of nursing advice at district level.

Both managers and nurses had great difficulty in defining 'nursing advice', and also the structure and instruments for collecting, disseminating and implementing such advice. Consequently, the transformation of the Chief Nursing Officer into the District Nursing Adviser as an add-on role, was viewed equivocally by both general managers and senior nurses alike. A role devoid of line management responsibility was unsatisfying to CNOs used to this power. The experience became mystifying, anxiety-provoking and extremely frustrating for some. 'Influence' over nursing had replaced 'control'. Ambiguity of status was seen by them to be their main problem.

By the end of 1988, only three of the original fourteen district CNOs who were in office in North West Thames prior to Griffiths were still in post. Two had left to become Regional Nursing Directors, and two had left their posts after a short period of appointment.

Those in quality assurance roles were also in a new field aimed at improving the services for the consumer, and impinging on many areas other than nursing. If the job were to be done properly it would take all their energies. At this stage, the nursing advisory function was felt by many to be a recognition that general managers wanted to have a nurse somewhere 'on call' at the district level, but that the 'advisory' role was being marginalised.

One DNA complained that when she went to a national conference attended mostly by general managers, a DGM remarked to her that the DNA role was 'useless', and indicated that general managers did not need pay too much attention to it. She said:

> He thought that I was a general manager, so he could say what he really thought about it. Quite frankly, I don't know how to explain my role to anyone. If I say I am a Director of a service, people understand, but advice is something too abstract, and not taken seriously.

Uncertainty about the exact nature of new roles affected recruitment. 'Influence' had replaced direct 'control' over nursing. Ambiguity of status was a major problem for those who remained in post.

A cycle of experimentation

Over the region as a whole, three CNO posts became vacant, in the first two years after the reorganisation, and no appointment was made for 6–12 months, during which time a DNS within each district acted up in the role. This proved problematic, particularly in the large teaching hospital districts where shortages, absenteeism, training issues and enormous organisational change were profoundly affecting the workforce. The DNS/DNA was placed in a difficult position. Unit commitments often conflicted with district level meetings and took precedence.

Some DNSs in this position were not supported by their peer-group, who felt that they did not need advice from a colleague who was an equal. Perhaps this attitude was an outcome of being socialized in an hierarchical system, both within nursing and in the NHS more generally. In some smaller districts, these DNS/DNA roles seemed to work better. As the local organisation was less complex, there was less pressure on the workforce and less structural change to destabilise relationships.

A common cycle was perceivable in the three districts where the CNO left (Fig. 6.2). General managers eventually reverted to making a district level appointment. After the experiment, they recognised the difficulty of performing district responsibilities from a unit level.

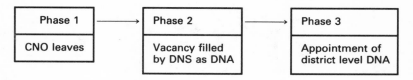

Figure 6.2 *Cycle of change in three districts*

Over the region as a whole, therefore, there was an unresolved and continuing debate about the proper place for 'nursing advice' between nurses and general managers throughout the 3-year project. The situation that had evolved by the end of this period is illustrated in Table 6.2.

The trend has been towards district level appointments with only two exceptions. It is fairly evenly spread over part-time DNA

Table 6.2   *Changes in NWT district level of nursing staff in 1985–8*

Changes in 14 districts		New roles	
Retired CNOs	7	DNS/DMS/DNA posts	2
In post	4	Part-time district DNA	2
Left for other NHS posts	3	Full-time DNA/CNO	4
		Full-time DNA/hybrid	5
Total	14	Total	13*

* 2 districts have fused into one

appointments, and full-time ones. The three districts that had opted for either a hybrid role, or no nurse at all at district level have since moved towards a more exclusively DNA type model.

National advice

The debate was not confined to North West Thames. It had been widely publicised in the nursing press. Our own first interim report (Glennerster & Owens, 1986) had discussed the issue as had a report from the Nursing Policy Studies Centre (Robinson & Strong, 1986).

In 1987, the Director of Regional Liaison at the DHSS warned regional general managers that, as part of the reviews, Ministers would monitor each region's achievements during the past year and 'nursing advice' would feature as a major item (Merifield, 1987). The letter began by saying that many felt that there was no problem, but as many nurses did, it was important to ensure that arrangements for getting good professional advice were as effective as possible. The letter then clarified what the DHSS considered to be the basic elements of the nursing adviser's role. They were:

● Input into operational and strategic planning and education policy;
● Monitoring the quality of nursing care;
● Professional leadership and performance assessment, setting professional standards and procedures;
● Acting as spokesperson on all nursing matters.

The letter set out a range of alternative roles that had been adopted by authorities reflecting some of the conclusions of our first report (Glennerster & Owens, 1986). These were as follows.

1 District Adviser as sole person.
   Individual DNAs can devote all their time to the post but their status is uncertain and they could lose touch with day-to-day practice.
2 District Adviser and Manager with other duties.
   The post holder is part of the general management team but has little time to do the nursing job.
3 District Adviser and UGM.
   Similar problems of time allocation arise, and individuals may find it difficult to concern themselves in the affairs of another unit.
4 District Adviser and Unit Nursing Officer (DNS).
   The post holder has 'hands on experience' but little time.

In short, the letter summed up the experience of North West Thames and other regions quite well, without resolving any of the problems or actually giving guidance. We were able to watch how some of these roles worked out in practice over two years.

District nursing advice in four districts

For a period of two years we observed the work of four DNAs at close quarters. Two researchers spent time with them in sample weeks following their pattern of work, attending meetings with colleagues, visiting units, and ordinary office hours. DNAs also kept a diary, which we analysed. The four district posts illustrated the variety of roles that DNAs were combining. They are set out in brief in Table 6.3.

Everyday life for a DNA

Far from the abstractions of DHSS circulars the everyday lives of a DNA were a complex interaction between the kinds of tasks set out in the DHSS letter, and the additional line-management tasks. The quality assurance role overlapped considerably with the task of monitoring and developing standards of nursing care. The DNA in District A was in this situation.

Table 6.3   *Hybrid roles for DNAs*

District	DNAs joint roles
A	Chief Nursing Officer Director of Consumer Services Quality Development
B	Chief Nursing Adviser UGM Community Service Director of Quality Assurance
C	District Nursing Adviser Director of Nurse Education
D	Unit Director of Nursing Unit Director of Inpatient Services 'Acting' District Nursing Adviser

The diary returns taken midway through the period of research showed that a large part of the work in this hybrid role had to be classified as 'shared work' (Table 6.4). Those DNAs who were main-line managers either as a UGM or a Head of Nursing Services spend most of their time on these pressing jobs, about 23–24 hours a week. It was only by working long hours that they managed to devote 13–17 hours to the DNA role. Because of the pressure these individuals were under, they gradually negotiated to appoint part-time assistants to relieve some of the daily burdens (Table 6.5), but this was on an *ad hoc* rather than planned basis.

Some DGMs opted to do without a DNA at district level at all. In three districts where this happened, after a period, sometimes up to a year without a nurse at district level, an appointment was made. At the end of 1988 only one district opted for a combined unit/district DNA role. All others appointments were at district level. Eight of the appointments are now full-time CNO/DNAs. Of the ten hybrid roles created during the research period 1985–8, only three remain. *This indicates that there is a return to the earlier system of a leading nurse at district level.*

The kind of pressures people in these posts were under can be illustrated in District D. As Head of Nursing Services, this person had professional responsibility for nurses working within a unit. This involved meeting fortnightly with Senior Nurse Managers

Table 6.4   *Support for the DNA.*

District	Role	Support staff
A	DQA/PS/CNO	Full-time Secretary (district level) Part-time Assistant for DQA/PS role

B	UGM/DNA/DQA	Assistant Deputy UGM
		Full-time Personal Secretary
		    (district level)
		Full-time Assistant DQA/DNA
		    (district level)

C	DNE/DNA	Full-time Personal Secretary
		    (district level)
		Full-time Assistant DNE
		Full-time Manpower Nurse
		Full-time Patient Care Developer/
		    Nursing Process Facilitator

D	Ass. UGM/ISM Acting DNA HNS	Full-time Assistant (district level) Full-time Secretary/PA (district level) Full-time Secretary ISM role Full-time Administrative Assistant

Table 6.5   *How DNAs spend their time*

District	Time spent in each role (h)			Total hours worked
A	DQA/PS 8 h	DNA 22½ h	Shared work 18 h	48½ h
B	DQA/UGM 24 h	DNA 13 h	15 h	52 h
C	DNE 24 h	DNA 19½ h	7¼ h	51½ h
D	ISM/HNS Assistant UGM 23 h	Acting DNA 17 h	14½ h	54½ h

Key: **DQA** – Director of Quality Assurance; **PS** – Patient Services; **DNE** – Director of Nurse Education; **ISM** – Inpatients Service Manager; and **HNS** – Head of Nursing Services

(SNMs), and with other support staff within units weekly, or in some cases daily. There were daily meetings with the assistant DNS's, individual meetings with Ward Sisters, and irregular meetings with general managers on operational issues. There were joint planning committees with local authorities, and attendance was required on multidisciplinary specialist committees on ethics, medical advisory matters, drugs and therapeutic groups, or AIDS strategy groups. The list of possible committees seemed endless.

To the duties that sprang from being responsible for nursing services in a unit, were added the district tasks. Nursing recruitment and levels of staffing shortage were constantly being reviewed. Nurse education was under regular discussion. There were complaints procedures and nursing disciplinary problems at unit and district level, draft papers for the DHA. It was necessary to sit on external committees, such as UKCC Professional Conduct Committees and Regional Advisory Special Committees, to conduct ENB approval visits, attend district meetings or clinical practice groups, assisting with senior appointments or chair committees at unit and district or regional level, attend and arrange meetings to discuss current topics such as Project 2000, and deal with the complexity of matters brought daily from the DHSS, the region and professional bodies for the attention of the DNAs in each district.

This list is not exhaustive by any means, but gives the general flavour of the demands made at unit and district level. The DNS/ DNA was also at a disadvantage being outside the DMB, and had limited capacity to attend all meetings expected as DNA. It was therefore more difficult to have a global view of the organisation. *Thus, for all those DNAs in dual roles in our study, the most difficult factor was getting the balance right between the different functions.* Those located within a unit structure had greater conflicts than those at district level. This was not altogether a conflict of interests, but a much more basic conflict in dividing time between the demands of the unit and those of the district. The appointment of assistant staff had eased this problems, but these were *ad hoc* arrangements.

The second most important factor for the success of the role was that the DNA was overtly supported at district level by the DGM. This had effects on the individual's self-perception and image in relation to colleagues, both outside and within nursing. Two out of the four DGMs displayed an ambivalent attitude towards the nursing advisory function and this undermined confidence. Another problem was that the nursing workforce tended to feel that DNAs ought to carry on as before, pressurising the DNA to act as Chief Nursing Officer in a situation where they could not do so.

The DNAs were anxious to keep the profile of nursing high and be seen as the leader of the profession, but the NHS as a whole had set itself the goal of allocating responsibility and authority downwards to nurse managers within the units, clinicians and Ward Sisters. A revolution had begun, but for those at the top it created tension and dissonance. They had professional responsibility but little real authority within the unit structures.

Creating a new role

In 1985, the National Audit Office had described the planning and control of nurse staffing as 'haphazard'. After 1985, the situation worsened in North West Thames as responsibility for handling the workforce became fragmented. Personnel departments and units took over partial responsibility, which before had been focused exclusively within the nursing hierarchy. In 1988, the *Nursing Times* (1988a) map of national nursing establishments and shortages revealed that the numbers of nurses working in districts were unknown in seven of the fourteen regions. In our own research, it took several weeks of work in the four districts to collate the nurse manpower figures in 1987. Two DNAs were unable to complete the district figures, but no doubt after the grading review in 1988 the real nature of the workforce and its size could be more readily ascertained.

Managers contended that they knew the figures, but at both regional and district level they had great difficulty in actually producing any detailed data. One DNA, when asked to produce some data on this subject, sent a copy of the staff returns for the whole of the midwifery unit – she literally had no other figures to send. Where detailed figures were produced for two districts in late 1988, there was no consistency in the presentation or analysis between districts.

Overall figures are very crude as they disguise specific shortages. District D had a shortage of 39 per cent in the psychiatric unit. Three intakes of students had been cancelled, because of poor

recruitment, and there were also serious shortages of other professional, technical and administrative personnel; this consequently
affected nursing. There were also major shortages in the nursing of
the elderly, which reflected the more general situation in inner and
outer London.

The figures are difficult to interpret because of the inclusion of
learners in some figures, and also maternity leave vacancies.
State Enrolled Nurses are not consistently treated. In short, the
picture is one of extreme complexity and there are several difficulties
in interpreting the available data. Professor Alan Maynard suggested that there was a lot of 'hogwash about nursing shortage' and
pointed out that little attempt had been made to actually evaluate
the workforce using computerised techniques to work out efficient
skill-mixes of staff (Maynard, 1987c). What he and others failed to
understand is that, in many Health Authorities, the responsibility
for nursing information had been diffused in the reorganisation
process. *There was no guiding force, no one in control.*

It was in this context that the DNA in District C sought to grapple
with the issue. In her view there were seven main problems to be
addressed:

1   The size of and nature of the workforce had to be ascertained;
2   A re-evaluation of establishment numbers was required using
    some consistent standards;
3   Cooperation of all UGMs had to be won;
4   Appropriate measures had to be introduced;
5   The introduction of IT at the middle-management and ward
    level had to be thought through;
6   The responsibility for organising a district-wide strategy then
    had to be recognised and the tasks allocated; and
7   There had to be resources to motivate and maintain staff.

A core group of DNSs was formed to address and take action on
key nursing issues, with recruitment and retention as a priority.
They operated as a team of equals, with one acting as a coordinator.
The DNA decided to bring all her information together. She had
inherited several posts at district level some of which were vacant
and which she quickly utilised. She was fortunate that they had
not been swept away at the outset. Her team had specific tasks to
gather information about the workforce. This was constituted as
follows:

1 Two nurses to perform regular evaluation of quality of care, using Monitor and Criteria for Care;

2 One nurse to systemise information on patterns of sickness and absence, assist visits to develop and utilise information by collecting information on:

    (a) Performance indicators

    (b) Ward statistics

    (c) Costs per bed per patient

    (d) Bed occupancy rates

    (e) Levels of dependency;

3 One nurse educator, accountable to the Assistant DNE, to implement the nursing process.

All information was regularly and systematically collated by the DNA and DNSs, and recommended levels of skill-mix were created to help UGMs reassess and adjust establishment levels, to facilitate delegation of nursing budgets to middle managers and, in some parts, to ward level. This was an ongoing process which had to be repeated annually. Situations were constantly changing and recommended levels were adapted. The ultimate effect was very positive.

In addition, the DNA initiated a review of nursing services in the district. Over a period of eight months, 214 nurses were interviewed and 290 questionnaires completed. One of the major constraints identified was the lack of appropriate information systems.

This district, in one unit, turned a £250 000 nursing budget deficit into a £130 000 saving. The main savings resulted from stabilising the workforce. Agency nursing costs were cut by 40 per cent. The saving on the nursing budget was re-invested into improving the working environment and quality of care, and not 'clawed back'. It is difficult to say that there is a precise logic in management structures, or that this model structure could achieve the same effect in another district. How much was achieved by the personal dynamism of this particular DNA cannot be measured but in a neighbouring district with a similar environment there was a 20 per cent shortfall of nurses, and this did not improve in the period of our research. This suggests that internal factors and leadership can produce results in spite of a hostile external environment.

This DNA created a two-year programme of in-service training for Staff Nurses, in order to enlarge their experience and encourage them not to leave immediately after qualifying. This meant persuading the DMB to provide extra resources for these extra training needs, which had to be costed and carefully planned before the money was forthcoming. This was difficult in a tight financial situation.

It can only be concluded that coordinating, developing and planning a strategy for nurse manpower requires a district-wide focus and strategy, and a team of staff with the time to do it. It requires managers with the capacity to lead, influence and encourage their nursing colleagues and general managers willing to support the endeavour. The DNA in these circumstances is *providing the tools to support good unit management.* This is a very different style of management, less authoritarian than of old. The manager is flexible and approachable, and acts as a planner and facilitator, rather than a controller. This DNA demonstrated that there is a role at district level that is valuable, that positively assists those at the ward and fieldwork level, and responds to their needs in a turbulent organisational environment.

Questions remain unanswered

A different pattern of events was observed in another district. Here the DNSs were so long without a district level appointment that when someone was finally appointed there was a feeling of group hostility. The nurses themselves felt that the post was unnecessary, and that most nurse-related issues could be resolved within the units, or professionally in the District Nursing Advisory Committee (DNAC) or its core group. What had happened here was that the DNSs had formed a power base, and were reluctant to return to the former Salmon-type structure, with professional authority emanating from on high. As a peer group they had come together, and formed close relationships. *But the problem of representation at district level remained unresolved*, as DNSs acting as the DNA were faced with the conflict of unit versus district business already described.

The DGM in these circumstances was not left alone to make decisions about the question of appointing a DNA, or the form that role should take. There was a considerable amount of outside pressure from regional nursing staff and professional bodies to press him to conform to a semblance of the previous order. In the face of the large-scale reorganisations that were to take place both in student nurse education and major hospital closures in the district, the DGM concluded that a district appointment should be made to oversee those changes.

The DGMs, UGMs and DNSs in this district all questioned the need for a DNA post. Yet in a district with a four-thousand strong nursing workforce and with shortages, there needed to be some way to pursue an active nursing manpower strategy, and to carry through the major changes that district policy imposed on the nursing workforce. An alternative argument was that the workforce in this district was too large for any one person to have an overall view, and that power to adopt the approaches used in District C should actually rest with the DNSs in each unit. *What these two cases illustrate is the different ways in which professionals can view the organisation in which they work.*

Nursing Advisory Committees

Prior to the Griffiths Report the Nursing Advisory Committees in each district consisted of a group that represented *all* levels of nursing with an elected chairman. After the Griffiths changes, these bodies in North West Thames had become composed primarily of DNSS. To some extent, this was a deliberate strategy to increase the strength of an hitherto, ineffective nursing organisation in the face of the Griffiths changes.

An important development of this system was that the Chairmen of those groups were in all but one case the DNAs who were appointed at district level, and not elected by members, as before. These DNAs sat on a *Regional* Nursing Advisory Committee (RNAC). This facilitated the transmission of information to and from the region which was of professional interest (Fig. 6.3).

The new structure formed a basis for informing the DNA of national and regional nursing matters. All correspondence and circulars concerning nursing from the UKCC, ENB, RCN and DHSS were also brought to these meetings at both levels, and discussed and disseminated. It provided a forum for exchange of information and ideas, but it also had the effect of forming a power base or a collective voice for nursing at district level.

General managers or speakers from other disciplines were rarely

Regional Nursing Advisory Committee
Chairman: Regional Director of Nursing
Members: 14 DNA

District Nursing Advisory Committee
Chairman: District Nurse Adviser
Members: DNSs from units

Figure 6.3   *The nursing advisory structure in North West Thames*

invited to attend these meetings. On the whole, they were very inward-looking, focusing mainly on training of staff, recruitment and service issues and reflected the preoccupations of nurse managers (Table 6.6). The figures show the principal topics discussed in each meeting.

Table 6.6 illustrates the high level of concern about recruitment. The main problem was that in the forum like the DNAC alone, these difficulties could not be resolved. The DNAC could not really act as a group. The creation of a policy for district-wide recruitment or retention was often impossible, because participants had only a general, and sometimes scant knowledge of the actual numbers of their own workforce.

As one nurse put it: 'There seems to be a sea of paper and a desert of information'. Certainly there was a deluge of information coming from all directions, strategies to be commented on, priorities being set by the region, DHSS circulars and joint statements of philosophy that had to be worked out – for example the treatment of patients with AIDS. In one DNAC, there was a general feeling of pleasure that the nurses had produced a philosophy and strategy for coping with AIDS before the medical staff. Yet a policy for nurses alone *indicated a parochial attitude* that ignored the need for a more general policy for all groups of health workers.

In short, these advisory committees were useful for discussing and transmitting the implications of regional policy, but if they were to be more than that, the DNA or a group of DNSs on the committee had to take an issue away and pursue it in depth. The line between unit matters and professional matters was very fine. The special-interest groups for the elderly, handicapped, mentally ill and so on, which were related to some DNACs structures, were not seen to be

Table 6.6 *The content of Nursing Advisory Committees: main
incidence of topics discussed at Nurse Manager and DNAC meetings*

Issues	Percentage of meetings at which these issues were discussed
Training issues	DNAC(%)
Basic	27
Post-basic	37
Management	37
In-service	11
Recruitment issues	DNAC(%)
Students	37
Trained Staff	11
Retaining Staff	37
Agency costs	34
Shortfalls	—
New posts	20
Staffing standards	40
Staffing levels	11
Skill-mix	3
Service issues	DNAC(%)
Aids	22
Drugs/Injections	68
Equipment/Supplies	25
Cleaning	6
Laundry	—
Catering	3
Blood/Laboratories	—
Portering	—
Communication	8

very active during the research period. This is possibly because unit managers were addressing these care group issues on a more multidisciplinary basis.

Summary

1 The post of DNA is still ill-defined and ambiguous. The principal ingredient for its success is overt support from general management to legitimise its existence and importance in the

organisation. It is essential to provide a positive role model for nursing.

2 The conception of the role has had to change. Leadership has had to move towards negotiation and influence rather than authority and control. This is more problematic in a system like nursing, which was based on a militaristic model.

3 The idea of a professional hierarchy with a 'boss nurse' dies hard and has led to some confused thinking. It is difficult for some nurses to accept the loss of a district level nurse as it has implications for their standing as a profession in the NHS and their power within the organisational hierarchy. Some younger nurse managers appointed since reorganisation take a different view. They welcome power being devolved downwards.

4 Information systems in nursing are critically important and largely lacking. Telford studies and dependency studies are not always used to improve the system. Often they are left merely gathering dust in an office. This happened in two districts. Today's service needs someone capable to take charge of this function. One district produced a systematic approach that was coordinated by the DNA at district level.

5 The sheer volume of the information generated at every level in the NHS means that the DNA is a key person to facilitate the flow between different levels of the structure.

6 The DNACs are useful forums for discussion between top professionals. Their capacity to act or initiate is limited. They are a focus for information dissemination, and this in itself is an important function in so large an organisation. The creation and updating of drug policies and so on are examples of processes that regularly need readdressing at district level.

7 'Action groups' to solve specific problems within units should be multidisciplinary in the future, as nursing issues such as AIDS actually relate to all care staff. A *joint* not professional unilineal approach is necessary.

7
Deconstruction and reconstruction

————————— ◆ —————————

The processes of the Griffiths reorganisation have involved a dramatic change in management philosophy, or as theorists would say, a change of 'culture'. This means that new shared values and perceptions have to replace earlier ones. The most fundamental change is the reversal of the 'top down approach' (Griffiths, 1983 (para. 12d)), and a movement away from functional management hierarchies (Griffiths, 1983 (para. 29)).

Griffiths identified the problem of over-organisation of line management structures, and challenged the idea that functional management was necessary from the region to the ward level. He wrote that the further away from direct patient care the manager was, the less important it was that that manager should come from a specialist background. This statement was suitably vague, leaving open the question of 'how far to go' in applying this logic within the units (Griffiths, 1983 (para. 16, p. 18)).

The early interviews with senior nurses within the units made it clear that they felt that the traditional career routes offered by the Salmon functional hierarchy to management and to positions of power in the organisation were now threatened. In an interview with a reporter from the *Nursing Times*, Sir Roy contended that the traditional career routes still existed in many Health Authorities (*Nursing Times*, 1987), and that this was indeed the case in some parts of North West Thames. However, the reality was that, even in those districts where conservatism prevailed, the pressure to change and conform to this new culture was strong.

The Griffiths Report had emphasised that there was no remit to change 'statutory structure, organisation or finance of the NHS ... the NHS is in no condition to take another re-structuring, and more can be achieved by making the existing organisation work in practice' (para. 35, p. 23). The report also suggested that the service was also over organised (para. 3, p. 10). A few UGMs adopted a 'wait and see' approach but, in the face of radical change elsewhere, the more cautious after three years were also introducing changes, and common patterns began to emerge across the districts.

The rate of change in unit structures not only differed from district to district but also within districts. For example, two acute units within a district could have entirely different management structures. Organisational patterns may change, but the beliefs, values and patterns of behaviour of staff may remain much the same. This was evident as our fieldwork progressed.

Nevertheless, as Gertrude Stein once remarked 'A rose, is a rose, is a rose . . .', the same could be said of structures. Essentially, the service remains the same in spite of changing structures. It could be argued that the nature of the Health Service, particularly in the acute sector, is defined by the technological base and size of the organisation. These are the major factors determining and constraining organisational design (Hall, 1977). Demanding change is not enough, generating commitment to a new philosophy is also important.

This chapter focuses on the unit middle managers. They carry the burden of re-orienting nurses from a unilineal disciplinary approach, to a more comprehensive conception of the service as a whole. The major problem for nurse managers is that they must first change themselves and their own attitudes. This is achieved by general management teams such as the Unit Management Board (UMB) of which the DNS will be a member, having regular meetings, or occasional working weekends away together. The UGM's major task is to get all his or her team pulling in the same direction and sharing the same values.

Inevitably, the process is a slow one. Districts have reorganised at different speeds. Some individuals have found the 'cultural change' more of a 'culture shock' and have left the NHS, or have been asked to leave. In addition, training programmes have been out of step with such massive shifts in management expectations and role requirements; this had also happened in the reorganisation of the social services in 1970 (Billis, 1984).

The pre- and post-Griffiths unit structures

In the typical pre-Griffiths structure, a district could have four or more units. Each unit had a Director of Nursing Services who was the line manager for the nursing staff (see Fig. 7.1). He or she handled all issues of professional discipline and standard setting, acting under the ultimate responsibility of the District Nursing Officer. As we saw in the last chapter, the line of responsibility joining the Directors of Nursing Service to the district level had gone, as all managerial accountability now lay with the UGM. What Unit General Managers had to decide was whether to leave the nursing line-management structures untouched or to pursue the general management principle downwards.

Some units were completely reorganised. Each was divided into district sub-groups of services with a 'mini' general manager responsible for each. One early version of such a pattern is shown in Fig. 7.2, which illustrates a typical large hospital. There were many other variants. As in an industrial organisation, it was possible to put a non-specialist general manager in charge of each sub-unit and give them full line-management responsibility. It was at this point that UGMS had to grapple with the issues raised in Chapter 4. How far could an assistant unit manager who was not a nurse handle issues of professional discipline and standards?

If these issues arose and could not be handled by a lay manager, a professional nurse from another part of the organisation would have to be introduced to advise or deal with the issue. Therefore, two people would be involved and each had dual responsibilities. In our interviews with senior nurses at the beginning of the research, *this aspect of dual accountability was a major source of anxiety* (Glennerster & Owens, 1986).

In Fig. 7.2 the possibility of such dual responsibilities was minimised because the Director of Inpatient Services, with the largest nursing component, was also a nurse and was given DNS status. She was responsible for handling professional issues that arose in the theatres and in the outpatient clinic and accident and emergency unit. This task involved considerable sensitivity because it meant invading the territory of the Assistant Unit General manager.

The structure illustrated in Fig. 7.3 gave rise to many more dual patterns of responsibility. Only one of the location managers was a

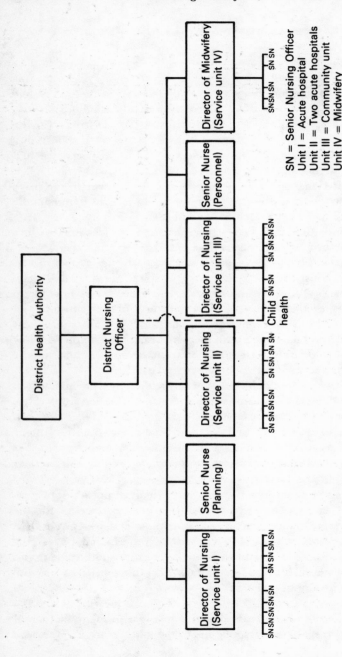

Figure 7.1 *Pre-Griffiths nurse management: where* ———— *= joint management/professional responsibilities and* - - - - *= professional issues*

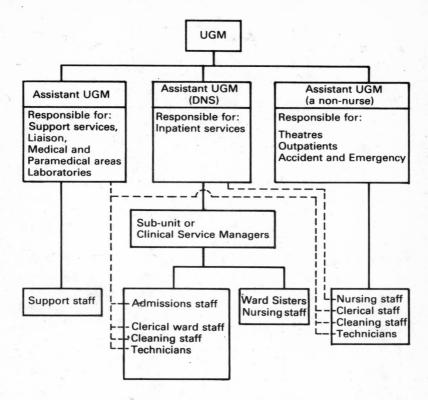

Figure 7.2 *A post-Griffiths unit structure: where* ____ = *line management;
and* _ _ _ _ = *professional responsibilities*

nurse who also had responsibility for handling professional disputes,
not merely in her own part of the service but in the other 'locations'
in the community unit.

Early in our research it became clear that there would be
problems associated with the separation of professional advice and
line-management functions. They were not frequent daily occur-
rences but when they happened they could be serious. Nevertheless,
it also became clear that the individuals concerned found ways to
cope. When the DNSs had to handle professional issues in another
part of the unit from their own, they usually did so with sensitivity.
Equally, general managers began to recognise that there was a real
issue here. The newer structures *minimised the extent of this conflict*

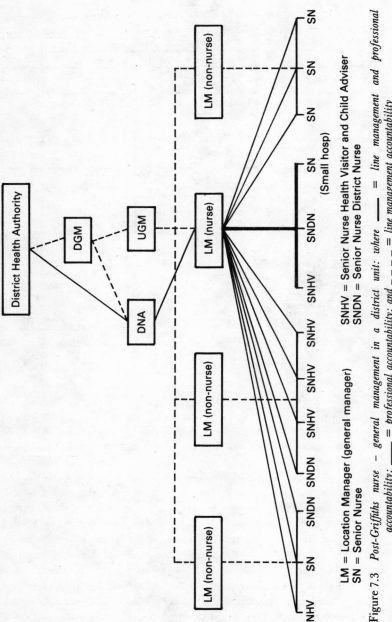

LM = Location Manager (general manager)   SNHV = Senior Nurse Health Visitor and Child Adviser
SN = Senior Nurse   SNDN = Senior Nurse District Nurse

Figure 7.3 *Post-Griffiths nurse – general management in a district unit: where* ——— *= line management and professional accountability;* ——— *= professional accountability; and* _ _ _ _ *= line management accountability*

by appointing nurses to manage those units where nurses were the largest part of the workforce, as in Fig. 7.2.

In the next section we illustrate the distinct professional issues that could arise.

Accountability and communication

In the former structures, there was a Director of Nursing Services (DNS) who was responsible for all nursing shifts within a unit (see Fig. 7.1). In the first year of the project, there was considerable discussion, both at a national and local level, about the issue of dual accountability that arose in the general management framework (Glennerster & Owens, 1986).

The accountability of nurses is multifaceted. The nurse is: (a) accountable to the employing authority; (b) professionally accountable in terms of established codes of practice; and (c) personally responsible in common law terms and, as such, can be prosecuted.

In the new structures the question of who is responsible and who needed to know became crucial, not least because of these legal issues of personal (that is, for the individual nurse), and vicarious (that is, to the employer) liabilities. Nurses, as the primary deliverers of direct care, are at high risk of making mistakes or falling below standards because of the especially personalised nature of their job. Performing intimate tasks for the patient, delivering drugs and therapy, and daily personal interaction makes them especially vulnerable. Two cases of maladministration of drugs in the research period made it clear that both professional and general management responsibilities were involved. Any serious case inevitably involves outside agencies (Fig. 7.4).

In both these cases, the DNAs were drawn in for professional advice after external agencies had become involved. In the first case, the DNA felt a need to be involved in the resolution of the problem, but the UGM did not agree. In Case 2, the DNA was anxious to push the resolution back to the unit but was involved by the general managers. In both cases, there was profound uncertainty about what responsibility senior nurses in the units actually had, and how far the UGMs were also prepared to go without involving district level staff. Also, in each case, the unit managers came to recognise that these situations should be handled within the units, and no

Management problem	Internal involvement	External involvement
Case 1		
Drug given to wrong patient	DNS UGM District pharmacist DNA Medical consultant	Coroner Police
Case 2		
Drug appropriated by nurse	DNS UGM DNA/DGM Medical consultant District pharmacist	Drug squad Professional representatives

Figure 7.4   *Examples of professional–management issues*

longer passed up the hierarchy as had happened before the Griffiths' changes. That put a heavier responsibility on the DNS or equivalent in each unit. Different UGMs and DNSs organised their own system for dealing with disciplinary matters. *By the end of the research period, most heads of nursing in each unit either sorted out the problems independently or, if necessary, in cooperation with the UGM.* They also learned that problems that affected nurses and their work had implications for other groups of staff such as general managers and doctors, and could involve outsiders such as the law and representatives of trade unions or professional associations. *The impossibility of isolating professional accountability from other dimensions of management that affect the whole service was also recognised.* A close working relationship between the DNS and the UGM was essential and tended to become increasingly formalised in regular unit team meetings.

However, in resolving these individual problems wider issues were involved. In Case 1 the policy for drug administration had not been followed, and in Case 2 the addiction problem of the nurse involved had not been recognised. If the district is to be viewed as a total entity, any strategies for coping with these types of problems in one unit had relevance for others. This is where the DNA and the District Nursing Advisory Committee (DNAC) had a role to play.

A case in point

One example may illustrate the general point. Several units in the district were desperately short of qualified nurses at night. Many patients were on intravenous infusions, which meant that qualified staff were having to spend most of the night attending to drug administration, leaving most other tasks to the unqualified nursing assistants. Here was a situation where medical technology had established patterns of care, and where junior doctors were passing onto the nurses some of the routine treatments.

The effect on a diminished workforce was considerable. Most nurses at night were reluctant to disturb junior medical staff who were also overloaded and on duty during the daytime, sometimes up to 100 hours per week. The DNSs in the acute units took this general problem to their DNA as it had a professional dimension, which, in turn, influenced the deployment of scarce resources of qualified night nurses.

The DNA approached the District Medical Advisory Committee (DMAC), and some adjustments were made across the board to drug administration routines, prescribing practices and sharing responsibilities between medical and nursing staff. Agreement was reached on a district policy so that staff were not left to resolve those problems on an individual level.

From professional to service management

Acute units

The sub-unit service managers were, on paper at least, responsible for the whole organisation of their area of service. In the acute units, it could be for theatres, outpatient, surgical, medical, geriatric, accident and emergency, maternity units and so on. In the Griffiths terminology, the service managers were 'in charge'. However, in reality, porters, cleaners and clerical staff usually had some external organiser as well, outside the sub-unit, and doctors were also still outside the system of accountability at the sub-unit level. In many districts, consultants' contracts were held at the regional level not at district level, unlike other categories of staff. So structural changes were more apparent than real, as they did not signify changed power relationships.

The DNSs who moved into hybrid roles in the acute unit structures were often appointed as assistant UGMs or hospital managers. The content and importance of their roles actually grew compared with expectations in 1985. Non-medical UGMs quickly expressed a need for a high-level nurse in the organisation, to act as advisor across the whole unit. They usually combined this role with direct responsibility for inpatient services or, in the smaller acute hospitals, the function of hospital manager. Most DNSs in this situation agreed that their new jobs were more fulfilling and interesting than before.

Community, psychiatric and mental handicap units

In the community and psychiatric and mental handicap units, the pace and structure of change also differed widely between districts. Some community units stayed with structures based on line management of occupational groupings, for example District Nurses, School Nurses, Health Visitors, dental workers and so on. There was a cautiousness, in some districts, in taking on the recommendations of the Cumberlege Report (1987), or opting for Location Managers on the lines of Service Managers.

In the four districts studied, one or other of the models described in Figure 7.5 were in operation. But, those using (a) and (c) are aiming eventually towards model (b). The major problem with a transfer from model (a) to (b) is that if there is an existing DNS, and he or she is not appointed as a Location Manager, there is really no place in the system for such an individual apart from an unsatisfactory 'advisory role'. This happened in Districts A and C, where the DNSs became marginalized once location posts were established. In this situation, there was strong pressure for the DNS to leave. If she or he was nearing retirement less pressure was exerted, but it was almost certain that younger DNSs would be redundant in the new structures, even though their contract with the employing authority remained. This meant that in some units there remained DNSs with limited managerial roles.

The problem of dual accountability hardly arose in the community units studied, which was not surprising as nearly the whole workforce was composed of nurses, and two out of the four UGMs were nurses. In the other two units, nearly all the major Location Managers or Care Group Managers were nurses. In these circumstances, one

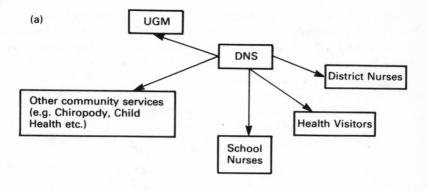

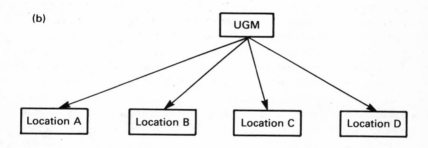

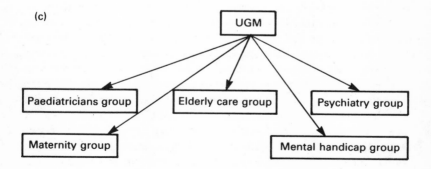

Figure 7.5 *Community unit structures: (a) traditional line management (community units); (b) location management; and (c) care group management*

manager was given responsibility for professional nursing matters throughout the unit.

Three structures exist in the community units (see Fig. 7.5). Only one non-nurse Location Manager was appointed, but this situation did not give rise to severe conflicts of professional versus managerial interests, although there were some signs of resentment and failure to cooperate by some of the district nurses. The continued existence of a DNS enabled the older system to persist, and this created confusion rather than conflict, as nurses were in the position of serving two masters.

There were tensions in the traditional systems too, as now the ultimate authority was the UGM, and even if that UGM was a nurse, the DNS found it difficult to defer to a higher authority, when formerly she or he had been that higher authority. Generally, the DNS in the community unit fared less well in the management stakes than colleagues in the acute units, as old and new patterns coexisted more uneasily.

The psychiatry and mental handicap units raised different problems. Here, as in the acute units, the DNSs in the four selected districts either became Assistant UGMs or Hospital Managers (HMs). Below them, a system of Service Managers and Ward Leaders/Managers was being developed, which reflected the changes at the top levels. Most of these posts were filled by nurses from the existing pre-Griffiths structure. The Hospital Manager/Nurse Manager role is comprehensive, covering service delivery and service development rather than exclusive responsibility for a professional group.

In the plans for mental handicap and psychiatric services, the policy is to return residents to the community. The HM has the dual role of maintaining and improving services within the existing institution, and developing a service outside it. This makes his or her role more varied and demanding.

To meet these objectives, new management training schemes have had to be elaborated. In one hospital, the ex DNS/new HM said that he realised that the nursing staff could not cope with too rapid a pace of change, and to enable them to keep up with the pace and adapt to new structures, change has had to be slowed down. Nursing staff in new Ward Manager roles needed training in budgeting and the introduction of Individual Care Plans (ICP) as a basis for future general management roles.

What's in a name?

We began by saying 'A rose, is a rose, is a rose', we could end by asking is all this renaming of nursing staff with general management labels simply 'a rose by any other name'? In other words, are the structural changes just changes in organisational taxonomy, disguising that underneath things are very much the same? We have concluded from observing day-to-day situations that in many respects this is the case. Clinical or sub-unit managers and ward leaders cannot actually be 'captains of their own ship'. Most of the non-nursing staff are not, in practice, under their direct control. It is true to say that the management training and systems necessary to make the real changes in organisational relationships were following rather more slowly in the wake of structural alterations of the organisation of the unit systems.

However, the processes of social reconstruction and deconstruction are not mere window dressing, they are the first steps in communicating by symbolic means the changing philosophy and culture of the NHS. These are the visible signs that 'someone is in charge', even if some would argue that it is merely like 'the mobile' changing position (to use Griffiths' own metaphor), and only an illusion. However, statements of facts can ultimately become self-serving truths.

Conclusions

1 The reversal of the top down approach began by making changes at the top in the North West Thames districts. It was not a uniform approach, as between districts and between units within districts UGMs adopted differential strategies. Some opted to maintain stability and the *status quo*, and others embarked upon radical reorganisation.

2 After three years it seemed evident that, in the acute units, a model based on hybrid roles for all managers of the direct care services was being created. A substantial pruning of middle managers, particularly nurses, occurred and a more simplified model of management developed. Most acute hospitals seemed to be moving towards a model of service management.

3   These structural changes were a first step in changing relationships and patterns of accountability in the units. Where a non-nurse was manager of a sub-unit, nurses had to refer professional matters to a Head of Nursing and to the general manager. This had the potential for confusion, but it was recognised that most problems were not one-dimensional as they affected the whole service.

4   It soon came to be accepted that one senior nurse manager was identified as professionally responsible for all nurses within each unit. Usually this person was a key nurse in the unit management structure as an assistant UGM or Hospital Manager in the acute, mental handicap or psychiatric sectors.

5   There were more variations in the community structures. Some opted for the traditional line-management model, others for care group or location-management models. In nearly all cases, these top management posts were filled by nurses. The DNSs who remained in the latter two models were marginalised, as they had no functions other than as advisers.

6   The hybrid roles at all levels imposed wider responsibilities for total service delivery and service development. However, the reality was that most relationships had not changed fundamentally. Doctors and ancillary workers, such as cleaners working for privatised companies, still operated as independent groups within the system. Service managers' authority over them was purely nominal.

7   In order to effect the changes in relationships, more education and training was necessary to change group loyalties from occupational ones to service ones, to create a more multi-disciplinary commitment within sub-unit structures.

8   The traditional career structure had been radically transformed for nurses but, actually, they occupied most of the unit Service Manager and key senior posts. The wider sphere of responsibility had, for most DNSs, enhanced their role in the organisation giving them more personal autonomy and a wider sphere of activity.

8
Conversion and confusion

————————— ◆ —————————

The previous chapter was concerned with the organisation of work over the Health Service units as a whole. This chapter moves down to what can be called *level three* work, which is always the most difficult to define and structure in any welfare organisation (Billis, 1984). This has certainly been true of nursing as discussed in Chapter 4, and has been observed by other writers (Kinston, 1987). In the last chapter, it has been suggested that there is a high level of dissonance between the images projected by the new structuring, the expectation of managers engendered by organisational change, and the reality of the experience for managers at middle levels of the units.

Drucker (1979) has suggested that level three management has to have authority for the security of the group. They are usually experts or 'knowledge workers', expected to protect workers from managerial ignorance, or alternatively to integrate workers into the mission, purposes and objectives of management. Increasingly, they can find themselves rejected from above and below. Nevertheless, 'No organisation can function if this level of management is not functioning, they are the connective tissue of the organisation.'

Over the last few years, there has been a major debate about the role of the senior nurse managers who work at this level. The two main criticisms of the old pattern have been that the Salmon hierarchy was overloaded and confused, alternatively that the posts were too oriented towards routine administration, and not enough to clinical support work. Nurses often compared themselves with the medical profession, but felt that promotion to management at this level meant that they lost out clinically, unlike their medical consultant colleagues. They felt that they lost touch with patients and merely became paper pushers.

Since the introduction of general management, the debate has moved on. The trend has been to give greater status and power to nurses at ward level, creating even greater uncertainty about what kind of work should be performed above ward level. The grading review in 1988, with large salary increases and seniority payments for Sisters, was the first step in this direction. It reflected the new general management philosophy to devolve managerial responsibility.

Where, if at all, did the Senior Nurse Manager (SNM) fit into this new scheme of things? Was there a case for a high-powered specialist clinician, an adviser with no line-management responsibilities? Should level three management, that is, the allocation of work priorities and so on, be undertaken by a service manager? If so, as some unit managers argued, that service manager did not have to be a nurse. In the early stages of the research these questions caused enormous anxiety and resentment among nurses at this level who saw their posts disappearing.

Yet, in the longer term, it was the absence of decisive change that caused the most concern. In those units where the changes we have just outlined occurred rapidly, the staff concentrated on reconstruction with a feeling of some foreseeable objective future and stability. In more traditional units, or those faced with closure or merger, continued uncertainty increased anxiety levels about personal futures, and created organisational inertia. It could be argued that the very open-endedness of Griffiths prescriptions at this level were responsible for this.

At the other extreme, some units seemed to be in a state of continuous change as managers oscillated between different notions of how to structure this level. New Unit General Managers (UGMs) needed to prove themselves. Organisational rearrangement was one way of appearing to be doing something. This atmosphere of endless possibilities was at once both stimulating and exciting for the new UGM but could be damaging and demoralising for those lower down the organisation as planning for the future at all levels was affected.

One middle manager who was not a nurse said, 'Since 1983, I have had four different changes in my job. I have not personally benefitted from the Griffiths changes, and I am thinking of leaving the NHS.' Actually, this complaint reflected the ambiguity that surrounded most middle-management roles. Unhappiness with the organisation of this level of management was not confined to nurse managers.

Historically, the intermediate status of the SNM had been an excuse for pushing decisions upwards. It could be said that the very nature of their in-between status meant that their ability to make decisions was constrained. Some critics have said that SNMs have rarely been held responsible for anything. As Billis (1984) remarked, titles of jobs and job descriptions say a lot about 'expected work' but tell us little about 'actual work'.

In one hospital, the number of SNMs was cut from thirteen to eight. In these situations, morale suffered as promotion prospects in nursing seemed to be disappearing.

In this chapter, three themes are addressed, namely:

- the devolution of power, authority and responsibility;
- defining service territories and roles; and
- creating a new career structure for nurses in NHS management.

Devolution of authority

In the four selected districts, we found quite different models of management at this level. A survey of nurse managers in nine acute hospitals revealed that they had three distinctive titles (Table 8.1). What was most striking about the groups as a whole was that, regardless of differing titles, very few of those middle managers were actually performing general management roles.

In spite of the rhetoric about devolving budgets to service or ward levels, this had only happened in a few service areas. Very few had total budgetary responsibility for anything other than for nursing

Table 8.1 *Middle-manager titles for nurses and numbers in nine acute hospitals*

Service Manager (SM)	14
Senior Nurse Manager (SNM)	16
Clinical Nurse Manager (CNM)	2
Total	32

personnel in their area. Clinical budgeting is the expressed aim in many districts but without the appropriate staff or information technology in place it is still a future prospect. Financial responsibility for supplies and equipment and other groups of staff was still fragmented throughout the units. Some discrete areas, such as midwifery and radiotherapy, lent themselves more easily to budget devolution.

The confusions are evident when, for example, staffing budgets are held by middle managers, and supplies and equipment budgets held by the DNS or assistant UGM. One Sister complained of being continuously berated for 'over spending' on supplies and equipment, but she had never been given an actual limit for the ward budget in spite of repeated requests. The nature of budget holding therefore is extremely randomised and idiosyncratic in the current structures, both old and new, which means that many managers are functioning in a veil of ignorance.

The authority of middle managers, therefore, was problematic. They were often accountable for spending within their sub-units, but apart from spending on the nursing budget, had little control over other areas of the Service. Nurse managers in our sample were responsible for a range of functions beyond nursing. Table 8.2 shows the percentage of managers who were responsible for several different service areas, which were often overlapping, giving wider responsibilities.

Table 8.2   *Middle managers group*

Service area	Middle managers responsible for this area (%)
ITU/CCU	31
Theatres	19
Surgery	31
Medical	34
A & E	12
Outpatients	12
Elderly care	16
Paediatrics	12
Other areas (e.g. Radiology and Dermatology)	25

No matter what the title, the essential nature of the job remained the same as before the Griffiths reorganisations. Most managers had a span of responsibility either for a specific department, or for three to six wards or for clinical work (87 per cent). A few (13 per cent) were covering a much larger span of work – seven to ten service areas for example (see Table 8.2).

When asked about their major focus of work in the previous week, no less than 63 per cent identified 'staffing the wards' as the principal task. Many complained that they were dominated by the day-to-day pressure to provide adequate nursing cover for their areas. The second major task was dealing with stress among nursing staff. Their third most time-consuming activity was to develop strategies for training and education of nursing staff.

In general, the major focus of all these roles was with the daily running of the service, and maintaining an adequate workforce. Out of the group, *69 per cent said that their actual roles differed little from those in the pre-Griffiths structure.* The major difference was that their formal responsibilities had been extended. There was felt to be an uneasy fit between the job titles and a realistic expectation of those roles.

Professional accountability was still to a head of nursing – the DNS. When asked to identify recent problems taken up the hierarchy, they too resembled the previous patterns. Disciplinary problems, staff sickness and matters affecting the recruitment or appointment of nursing staff were the subjects that ranked highest.

These areas of concern were often interrelated. *Disciplinary hearings were regularly associated with chronic poor work attendance, and shortages were consistently due to absences of staff as well* as shortfalls in establishments. In summary, the major areas of activity for middle managers were *still focused on purely nursing staff issues* and nursing activity, rather than on general service management.

Defining service roles and territories

Service Managers

One of the difficulties of achieving this change of role was that many SNMs had merely had their roles extended to that of Service Manager in the same unit. This lead to the familiar difficulty of redefining established relationships. DGMs who were ex-administrators, CNOs who became DNAs, DNSs who were transformed into hospital managers in their own units or districts, all experienced this painful process. One SM who had been the SNM said:

> Sisters still see me in the old Nursing Officer role and have little perception of what SMs do or should be doing. Because of the current nursing climate, I spent a lot of time sorting out every day running of the nursing service. This initially caused me frustration as it prevented me getting on with other management tasks. Clinical matters also dominate my service as I am continually sorting out premedications and other problems on the wards, and the bleep is continually going. I have no budget yet. I took this job as I thought it would generate less conflict than my last one in a London teaching hospital. I welcomed general management, but the reality is not that much different. The medical staff resent me enormously, they do not want anyone interfering in what they do. I feel I spend all my time sorting out staffing problems, which is always on a knife-edge of adequacy, and it's very difficult to do anything else.

This interview highlights the commonly articulated view that their work is dominated by daily administrative problems not the long-term work this level should be concerned with. Another major difficulty is that of convincing the medical staff that service management actually includes them. Old doctor/nurse relationships of dominance and submission have to be modified. In one unit, the UGM tried to encourage the doctors to become Service Manager. The discussion went on for nearly a year, and the doctors finally refused to take on the work when they realised what it would involve. Subsequently, three nurses were appointed, but one doctor openly refused to accept the senior status and authority of the SM and said so. This made a nonsense of the theory of sub-unit control by a single manager.

Failures of communication that result from doctors' reluctance to take the Service Manager's role seriously can have dramatic results. In one hospital, the suicide of a confused patient prompted an inquiry. The doctor who admitted the patient had failed to inform the Service Manager or nursing staff of earlier suicide attempts and had treated the patient as a medical problem. *Lack of real authority and control is the commonest complaint.* Some general managers thought that nurses were too preoccupied with the issue of control. But it was difficult to make any decisions to change staffing levels or staff mix, or shift financial resources from equipment to staffing or vice versa, in a situation where there was no clear financial responsibility at the service management level. One CNM remarked, cheerfully:

> Well, they keep changing my job, but its really just the same. . . . I keep forgetting my latest name! We're still managing the beds, the staff, supervising the domestics, and keeping everything going out of hours. I'm still working to my 1982 job description . . . I really don't know if I've got any real managerial clout.

Her job description actually reads: 'To coordinate so far as possible, the management activities of work carried out within the unit, between units and between disciplines', but, as she commented, 'it's hard to coordinate these things – especially with doctors who themselves feel in control and superior to middle managers'.

Senior Nurse Managers

Typically, over the three years of the research, Senior Nurse Managers who retained their purely nursing role nevertheless had to manage more wards and to cope with major change as well. Bed or ward closures were a case in point. Closure of beds had to be negotiated between middle managers, doctors and the UGM. There was evidence of a more flexible attitude developing between the unit managers and medical personnel, particularly in areas where staff were in short supply and where patients need high levels of individual care, but the middle manager had to play an important role. On one such ward for bone marrow transplants, the middle-manager saw her primary task as negotiating a reasonable balance of work that her nurses could sustain, with the admission policies of doctors. She said:

> It is my job to negotiate with medical staff on admissions, otherwise the nurses would crack, or turn to drugs or make

mistakes. At the same time, we must support the doctors in their
work of breaking new ground in order to help patients in the
future. We must all agree to admit some cases who are very
likely to die in spite of all medical interventions.

This SNM was very involved in actively supporting her staff at
the clinical level. During the processes of reorganisation, her sphere
of responsibility was doubled from 40 staff to 70, with 130 beds. She
felt that the quality of her work suffered as she spent most of her time
on the telephone staffing the wards. She left after only a short period
in this new extended role, for a more defined and less pressured job
in another hospital.

Clinical Nurse Managers

These managers had even greater territorial difficulties. They were
meant to act at ward level as a clinical backup for Sisters and nurses
as well as administrative backup. However, this caused difficulties
in defining what was the Sister's role in relation to the CNMs. They
often felt that they were treading on each others toes. In one
teaching hospital, in addition to CNMs, there were SMs as well,
creating *two* tiers of management between the DNS and Ward
Sister.

In these circumstances, both the CNM and SM complained of
difficulties in defining their separate spheres of responsibility, if
indeed this were possible. It was a situation that added to confusion
at ward level about who was in charge. The SM had budgeting
responsibility for the sub-unit, and the CNM was responsible for
recruitment and allocation of staff. The main complaint from the
CNM, was one that was echoed everywhere, 'the job is top heavy
with administration, and consequently lacks the clinical input', it
was therefore unsatisfying.

In this situation the SM had satisfactorily off-loaded the more
arduous and daily tasks to the CNM, in order to be able to get on
with the task of supporting and developing staff training and
planning for the Service as a whole. The delegation of routine tasks
seemed a sensible strategy but it was questionable, whether a skilled
CNM should be wasted as an administrator in this way. It suggested
that an administrative assistant would have been a better way of
achieving the same result.

There were also frequent complaints about the quality of the personnel services. It was claimed that they often lost application forms, were slow in following up applicants, and did not inform interviewees of the outcome of interviews in some cases. In many hospitals, efforts had been made to by-pass the personnel department by recruiting learners before they qualified. But these perceived failures in other departments added to frustration of middle managers grappling with major and persistent shortages.

In one sub-unit with many specialised services, there were 50 vacancies out of a staff of 172. The unit was characterised by high budgets, high dependencies and high staff ratios. This service was dogged by increasing levels of stress, expressed by staff who were constantly threatening to leave. The situation was exacerbated by the introduction of new medical techniques requiring more intensive nurse input, for example new dialysis procedures. The role of the middle managers here was one of constantly supporting staff and adjusting workloads. To ease the burden on middle managers, a Recruitment Officer had been appointed to take on some of the more onerous administrative pressures and to create a more ordered approach to the problems of recruitment and retention.

Making it work

In spite of the problems we have described, some units were devising structures that the staff felt were working. For example, we found one radiotherapy unit where the SM was a doctor, who had budget-holding responsibility for the Service. This SM had two assistants, a CNM and a Senior Radiographer who ran inpatient and outpatient services respectively.

The self-containment of this sub-unit was its strength. The doctor (SM), nurse and radiographer formed a team of managers who had control over the sub-unit budget, staffing ratios and admissions. There was a high level of consensus between them about the running of the unit. Some problems arose concerning the autonomous nature of the unit, which was situated in a hospital under continuous pressure for beds. The use of empty beds for patients with needs other than radiotherapy and cancer treatments, created tensions among staff.

A high turnover of staff occurred, particularly at times when more patients with terminal disease were admitted. Sisters changed every two or three years. The staff consisted of about 45 WTE and five Sisters, so much of the CNM task was supportive, and was concerned with the development and training of nursing staff. The work of the unit had changed substantially over recent years. New chemotherapy treatments to be given by nurses needed high levels of skill and training to administer complex and labour-intensive schemes. This CNM's task was well-defined and satisfying. She said: 'I am very happy in this job, I don't want to go anywhere else. The Service is always developing and I am never bored.'

The essentials in this job were that responsibilities were clear, there was a control over the budget for the Service as a whole, allowing for flexibility in resource allocation, and there was shared control. The key professionals organised themselves into a team to resolve problems and develop the service, doing away with the doctor–nurse paramedical divide, which colours so much decision-making. It was an illustration of the theoretical case for clear delegation of authority, and collaboration in small units that were discussed in Chapter 4.

Similar situations occurred in the areas where close working relationships were fundamental to the smooth running of the service; arguments about lists overrunning had to be resolved, because extra staffing costs adversely affected budgets. However, in two theatre sub-units SMs had been appointed by default because of long-term sickness of a colleague or lack of suitable applicants when the post was advertised. In both cases, the SMs had no training in managerial skills. One SM remarked, 'I'm too busy to think about training', while another remarked, 'It would all be too much after a busy day in theatre.' Nevertheless, in general, the lack of training for these new responsibilities was keenly felt, together with a lack of support from higher management.

Who are the middle managers?

In our sample 75 per cent of nurse middle managers were female. The length of time taken to reach middle-management level was, to some extent, dependent on family commitments. A high proportion had qualified over 20 years ago (Table 8.3).

The extent of instability at this level is suggested by the fact that

Table 8.3   *Careers of nurse middle managers*

Years from Sister to middle manager	
0–5 yrs	6%
6–10 yrs	47%
11–15 yrs	25%
15–26 yrs	22%
Dates of qualification	
1950–60	25%
1961–70	40%
1971–80	35%
Years in present posts	
1 year or less	53%
2–5 years	28%
6–10 years	19%

over half the group had been in post for one year or less, which indicated a large number of people grappling with new roles and responsibilities. All were recruited from SNM ranks, with the exception of one Sister who was acting up and felt overwhelmed and was longing for the day she could return to the ward. This was mainly because she lacked training and experience.

Most middle managers had attended some management training courses, 28 per cent had diplomas or degrees, but mostly they were trained by short in-service courses. When asked about future career plans their answers were mixed (Table 8.4). Nearly one third of the group saw themselves in general management roles in the future;

Table 8.4   *Future career directions*

General management	29%
Clinical nurse management	19%
Remaining as SNM	34%
Health care outside NHS	6%
Retirement	6%
Other role (e.g., Counsellor)	6%
Total	100%

this indicated that, in spite of all the difficulties, the principles of general management had been accepted by many middle-manager nurses. It is to be accepted that in the face of so much change, an equal proportion opted for the *status quo*, but a substantial proportion wanted to move towards a more highly technical or clinical specialism.

Community, psychiatric and mental handicap units

It is difficult to discuss middle management in these areas as each of the four selected had opted for different models of service. Location managers in the community units eliminated any higher authority in nursing, such as the DNS, thus compressing the hierarchical structure. They related directly to the field staff level. Community units opting for a care group structure also eliminated DNS. Each care group was managed by a separate individual performing level-three tasks. This makes comparisons with the acute units difficult.

In the mental handicap units studied, a movement towards nurse/hospital manager and nurse/ward managers with service managers in between was a reflection of the earlier system but, as with the acute units, it was accompanied by a philosophy of a more comprehensive management responsibility for 'a service' rather than a particular discipline.

Summary

1   The nurse middle managers in our sample in the acute hospitals had experienced major changes. Units were being restructured to eliminate pure nursing structures based on an occupational hierarchy, to ones that were based on a decentralised organisation.
2   The process of change had been different throughout the nine hospitals. However, even the more conservative units were now moving towards a Service Manager model, which suggests there will be more conformity in future structures. The new structures had dramatically reduced earlier SNM roles by more than half in most cases. This had not only substantially changed the middle-management role, but narrowed the entry gate to middle management.

3   Nevertheless, many of these changes were, as yet, present in name only, as reallocation of budgets for a whole service has only happened in a few cases. Mostly middle managers, whatever their title, were dominated by the task of staffing their wards and by responsibility for the nursing budget. They felt overtaken by the administrative role, which excluded or limited much clinical involvement.

4   This aspect has led to diminished job satisfaction for some managers. Their spheres of responsibility had been extended and therefore *increased* the staffing work. Responsibility for around 50 qualified staff seems to be the optimum acceptable. Over that figure, middle managers complained that their task became routine.

5   Some difficulties that staff identified were:
   (a) lack of preparation for those extended roles with further training;
   (b) jobs that nurses felt were too large to handle – they constantly felt inadequate; and
   (c) frustration at being overwhelmed by administrative tasks, and unable to be more active clinically.

6   Service Manager roles were not felt to be a reality unless, firstly, the budget-holding for the service as a total sub-unit was known, giving control and flexibility in deploying resources. Secondly, doctors had to accept SM roles, without which, control over resources was ambiguous. Doctors' non-acceptance of the role was based on former relationships between doctors and nurses, which had to be modified or reversed.

7   Nursing issues were still the major part of service management at this level and, consequently, most SM roles were filled by nurses. The older hierarchical structure still shadows the newer SM models, as disciplinary matters, the development of nursing policies, and other issues concerning training and staff development have to be synchronised and dealt with on a unit-wide basis. The professional hierarchy therefore continued to exist, albeit in a modified form. Similarly, other occupational groups, for example, the cleaners and porters, are accountable to other managers but there is no reason why this should not change, and each sub-unit should be responsible for its own staff of all descriptions.

8   The fragmentation of nursing personnel services and the

inadequacies of personnel departments were seen to be major
problems. Middle managers are dominated by these issues and
by the daily running of the service. The whole system needs re-
appraising. Either more support staff are necessary to lift the
administrative load, or a centralised system needs to be developed on each unit to deal with the needs of the services.
Giving Sisters their own responsibility for staffing is a further
option, and will be discussed in the next chapter.

9   A considerable amount of ambiguity surrounds the role of the
middle manager. SM structures give nurses in those posts a
hybrid role, greater power and responsibility in theory, but not
in reality in many cases, as there are so many constraints.

9
Pressure and change at ward level

———————— ◆ ————————

This chapter discusses the level of the Ward Sister or ward leader. The grading review became a national political subject of some importance in 1988 but the basic issues that it was trying to grapple with were of long standing. They derive not least from changes in the role of women in society as a whole. By the early 1970s it had become clear that Sisters could be expected to be in post for only relatively short periods. On average, they remained in a job for between one and two years before marrying or having a family. More opportunities for travel and work abroad, as well as more mobility within the population in general also underlay this change in employment patterns (Armstrong, 1981).

A study of nurse employment suggests that any analysis of labour turnover in nursing must consider the wider orientation to work within the structured constraints imposed by society. The view that stability in this labour force is mainly associated with high job satisfaction and vice versa is too simplistic. Women's priorities between work and non-working life play a major part, but even in the late 1970s there were signs of 'disenchantment' among nurses, mainly in relation to the system of rewards, comparative status and job satisfaction (Mercer, 1979).

Both the Pay Review Body (1988) and the Price–Waterhouse report (1988) suggested that there were deeper concerns in relation to management and heavier workloads, which we discussed in Chapter 3. In an attempt to enhance the value of the Sisters' role and the interest of the post, various experiments had been undertaken. In the Oxford DHA, a new structure was developed in the acute hospitals so that a senior Sister acted not only as manager of her own ward, but also as adviser and manager to two

Sisters-in-charge of other wards. The Nursing Officer (NO) posts were swept away, and instead new Clinical Practice Nurses were appointed in each unit to strengthen the clinical aspect of ward work. An internal performance-related pay structure was also introduced as an incentive to innovate. The effect of these changes it was claimed was to lengthen the average time a Staff Nurse stayed from 6–18 or 6–24 months, and more nurses were attracted to the units to work (Pembrey, 1980). Another variant was tried in Nottingham, where a UGM developed a simple three-tier system of UGM, Service Managers (SMs) and Ward Managers (Pickering & Fox, 1987).

Ward Managers were mini SMs responsible for every aspect of work in the ward except the clinical aspects of medicine. The training of these managers focused on: (a) encouraging a system of shared values; (b) budgeting, motivating staff, and communicating; and (c) adopting a tight-loose approach in terms of allowing Ward Managers to set their own standards, and monitor their own staff. There was surprisingly little resistance to the structural changes among the 'other staff' such as domestics and in catering.

In the North West Thames region research areas, change at this level has been less radical and slower. The top-down approach has been commented on in other chapters. It has meant that the perception of the organisation held by most Ward Sisters and Charge Nurses has been affected primarily by what has occurred in terms of restructuring the SNM tier.

The introduction of ward management in one mental handicap unit in North West Thames was in its early stages, and therefore could not be commented on. Additionally, the introduction of location managers in the community units was also in its early stages. It was therefore decided to concentrate on an in-depth study of 50 Sisters and Charge Nurses chosen at random in nine acute hospitals to complement the SNM/SM interviews, reported in the previous chapter.

Interviews focused on the Sisters' relationship with middle managers, and the kinds of issues that were taken up the hierarchy. Sisters also were given the opportunity to comment on workloads, morale and quality of working life. No direct questions were asked about the abstractions of working life such as stress or commitment to nursing or the NHS, but unprompted comments on these aspects were noted. The main findings are outlined in the following sections.

Table 9.1   *Characteristics of Ward Sisters*

Clinical areas	Percentage
Surgery	24
Medicine	20
Elderly	12
Theatres	10
A & E	12
Outpatients	4
Paediatrics	4
ITU/CCV	8
Other (e.g. Day Ward)	6
Total	100

Time in present post (years)	Percentage
0–2	46
3–4	22
5–6	12
7–8	6
9–12	8
14–16	6
Total	100

Time from qualifying to becoming a Sister (years)	Percentage
2–3	24
4–5	38
6–7	16
9–10	6
12–13	6
15–20	4
22–25	6
Total	100

Date of qualification	Percentage
1950–9	12
1960–9	26
1970–9	38
1980–8	24
Total	100

Characteristics of the group

Of the Sisters and Charge Nurses in the selected group 94 per cent were female and came from a variety of clinical areas (Table 9.1). A high proportion, nearly 50 per cent, had been in post for less than two years. About a quarter of the group had taken three years or less to become a Sister. These results were uniform across all the clinical areas selected in the four districts. It seems as if the shortages in nursing are accelerating the careers of some Sisters and creating a younger managerial group than before – a development commented on by others (Plant, 1985). Correlating the data on qualifications with type of district, it can be seen that more younger Sisters were located in the inner-city districts.

Staff and budgeting responsibility

Sisters were asked if they had responsibility in the new organisational structures for staff other than nurses. The situation of informal authority persisted for technicians, ward clerks, cleaners, porters, and so on. *It was strongly felt by some Sisters that cleaners should be part of the ward team and subject to their authority.* In the case of cleaning, there were consistent complaints about the low standards of service and lack of personal commitment to ward areas.

Only 18 per cent of Sisters had budgeting responsibility. Most had no idea of the budgets for their wards, this was located at the Service Manager level or above. The fact that 82 per cent had no power over the workforce budgets prohibited the changing of established patterns to suit needs. Many Sisters expressed a wish to have more control. However, only about half those interviewed had performed any dependency studies in the last 24–36 months, most establishments (90 per cent) were fixed, and were based on traditional figures. In these circumstances, *the most frequent complaint was that the workload had changed but the workforce had not.*

Out of contacts with Service Managers or SNMs made on the most recent meeting preceding the interview, 36 per cent were concerned with shortages of staff. Nearly half those interviewed had seen the SM/SNM that day, and 94 per cent within the last five days. Nevertheless, 65 per cent said that they were fully staffed according to agreed levels but that the most common cause of shortages were sickness or other absences. *Nearly half the group complained that they had major and chronic staffing problems resulting from sickness, absences or long-standing underestablishment.* The reasons for this lay in an absence of any really objective system for assessing staff requirements.

Relationships with SM/SNMs

Sisters were asked how they perceived the SM/SNM role. A very high proportion (48 per cent) perceived it as an almost exclusively administrative job. It should be emphasised that Sisters were never asked to comment about the personality of the SM/SNM involved but about the job itself. Many expressed sympathy for middle managers, typically commenting, 'they are desk-bound', 'they are simply running an agency service, stocking the wards with staff'. These comments mirrored the feelings of middle managers themselves. Many Sisters felt that contacts between levels of management were only about 'surface problems', or primarily concerned with staff shortages (Table 9.2).

'*Clinical problems*' *were rarely concerned with treatment issues.* More often clinical expertise was called upon to determine whether staffing levels would cope with additional admissions of highly-dependent patients, or for administrative back-up if the Sister felt it

Table 9.2 *Ward Sister–middle manager interaction: the principal issue discussed with middle manager at last meeting*

Staffing levels	36%
Clinical problems	22%
Career development	12%
Laundry, supplies & equipment	10%
Discipline/patient complaints	8%
Personal problems	4%
Disputes with medical staff	4%
Cleaning issues	2%
Other	2%

was necessary to close beds if there were too few staff available, and safety levels were threatened. Well over half the contacts between middle managers and Ward Sisters were concerned with the various aspects of having enough staff to do the necessary work.

Supplies and equipment and laundry services were frequently pushed up to middle-management level or higher, where budgeting control was located. Laundry services in some hospitals were a problem that took up far too much time at both the ward and middle-management levels. Several wards were changing some nursing auxiliary (NA) posts into 'housekeeping' posts to ease the burden of constantly badgering inadequate services; in some cases this was unsuccessful and ward clerks were needed to take on this role.

In one hospital with an in-house laundry, failure to equip and recruit laundry staff were the basic problems. In these circumstances, Sisters felt helpless to effect any change. In another hospital, using a private contractor, a breakdown in machinery led to serious shortages and high levels of frustration and anger. This bad feeling was pushed up to the middle managers who then vented their own feelings on the DNS, who then took it to the UGM. Problems like this and requests for equipment were still constantly pushed up the management hierarchy.

Sometimes it was felt that middle managers were being asked to 'rubber stamp' requests from the wards, or were simply double checking, and that is was a waste of managers' time. This was, to some extent, inevitable as few Sisters had control over budgets, and were therefore unable to make independent decisions about equipment and supplies. They were told by middle managers if they had overspent, but if they did not know where the budget was set it was difficult for them to assess spending.

A frequent, spontaneous complaint about middle management was that there was no system of appraisal of performance. There was no direct question in the interview about appraisal systems, but 20 per cent of informants mentioned the lack spontaneously. However, *only 14 per cent of Sisters themselves referred to any system that they personally conducted to appraise their own ward staff.* This group, in particular, felt that feedback from management was too often negative, and an absence of any staff evaluation system meant that positive reinforcement of good work done, and high achievements of staff was sadly lacking.

Future career

When asked about their future plans, about half the group expressed a preference for a clinical career, and were keen to explain that they did not aspire to the 'desk-bound' administrative image of some middle managers. Nevertheless, about *a quarter of the sample were willing and enthusiastic to move towards general management roles*. It was surprising that only 2 per cent wanted to go into teaching that was not ward based, although 46 per cent had attended short courses that would enable them to teach student nurses at the bedside. This seemed to indicate that the academic aspect of clinical nursing was the least popular career option.

Nearly half the Sisters had undergone some post-qualifying courses of a short-term nature. A very small number had not attended any courses. One Sister in the sample who had been in post for 14 years and who had attended no clinical or managerial updating courses was an exception. Of the group, 6 per cent had already obtained degrees. Only 12 per cent of interactions with middle managers were about staff development of Sisters.

Changes at ward level

One of the most significant changes affecting 36 per cent of Ward Sisters was the introduction of on-call responsibility, in rotation, for the whole hospital. Although some Sisters enjoyed the extended responsibility and new experience that this system offered, for many it was an additional burden that they found difficult to sustain. Out of the group 66 per cent complained of increasing workloads, and the bleep-carrying aspect was a dimension of this workload factor.

The workload factor was difficult to identify. Many Sisters complained that they filled in forms concerning dependencies or had done Telford exercises, without receiving any feedback or change or challenge to the status quo in staffing mix or levels. The general feeling was that this information was simply 'swallowed up by the management machine'. This explained the apparent contradiction in information about staffing and workloads:

● 62 per cent complained of increased workloads;

- 46 per cent complained of chronic, qualified-staff shortages owing to a variety of factors including sickness;
- 54 per cent were up to agreed establishment levels; and
- 44 per cent had performed some dependency study in the last two years.

It can be deduced from these findings that there are few systems operating in the acute units that efficiently, systematically and regularly serve the staffing requirements in clinical areas. For this reason, changing pressures in clinical areas are not assessed in any other way than by traditional 'rule of thumb'. The general picture that emerges is one of the middle manager attempting to treat the 'diseases' of low morale and high sickness and turnover rates of nursing staff, and consistently failing to take preventive steps to assess needs in a systematic way and to adapt staff levels and staff mix accordingly.

It is not always possible to obtain adequate nursing staff, but some wards were caught in a vicious circle of shortages because establishments had been set on some historical basis, which, by their very inadequacy, overloaded staff. *Using systems like 'Criteria for Care' it was possible to create a basis for correcting such imbalances in the staffing structure.* This required an initial expenditure in information technology and staff training but ultimately produced a more effective use of resources.

Of equal importance to these nurses was a regular and effective way of providing positive feedback to the nursing workforce about their performance and value. The effect of positive reinforcements is discernable in District C's system, which rewarded high perform- ance in clinical areas and actively involved the ward staff in the management process.

The 28 per cent of Sisters/Charge Nurses interviewed who spon- taneously referred to the low morale of their ward staff, were all too often in a situation where they felt their work was not valued or even recognised by higher management. In spite of these findings, it was noted that only 4 per cent of the group said that they actually wanted to leave nursing altogether, although a further 6 per cent said that they were considering nursing outside the NHS. In spite of all the stresses and strains, commitment remains strong to nursing in the NHS, and to the work of the Ward Sister.

Summary

1   About half the Sisters in the sample had been in post for only two years or less. This situation reflects a pattern that had become established in the early 1970s. It does not necessarily indicate a lack of commitment or high level of job satisfaction due to recent changes.

2   The restructuring of acute units had impinged on the Sister's role only minimally. Only 18 per cent had any budgeting responsibility at ward level, the majority had no control over resources and were acting in a supervisory role rather than a management one.

3   Most Ward Sisters/Charge Nurses complained that their establishments were set by tradition, and did not change even when dependency studies were performed. A lack of communication and responsiveness from middle management, and a feeling of having no control or capacity to change anything were common complaints.

4   Most issues discussed with middle managers were of an administrative rather than clinical nature. Over half the wards were staffed up to agreed traditional levels, but chronic sickness and absences were the core of discussions about shortages with higher management. These responsibilities were consistently pushed upwards.

5   Most of the irritations of ward management were off-loaded onto the middle managers, who were then at the interface dealing with staff shortages on wards, inadequacies in support services, and budgetary overspends. The SNMs, SMs and Clinical Nurse Managers are thus dealing with many 'second-hand' problems, thus duplicating management effort.

6   An absence of positive reinforcement for work well done, or recognition of staff commitment and achievement by middle and top management was felt to be a feature of relationships at ward level. Only 12 per cent of interactions with middle managers concerned staff development or training issues.

7   Around two thirds the group complained of increasing workloads, but this was related to their inability to actually adjust or change establishments. Additional responsibilities were associated with 'acting-up' in middle-management roles, and

being responsible for staffing across the hospital. For those Sisters/Charge Nurses on surgical wards with peaks and troughs of activity, it was difficult to take on this extra task.

8　In spite of these dissatisfactions, only 4 per cent of the Sisters wanted to leave nursing as an occupation, and only a further 6 per cent were considering working in the private sector.

10
Subjective and institutional arenas: the ward

———————— ◆ ————————

This final chapter allows the Ward Sisters interviewed to speak for themselves at greater length and describes some of the common problems that confronted nurses at this level. But these problems have a complex chronology and are of a long-standing nature. Griffiths has not necessarily addressed these issues. All the external forces referred to in Chapter 2 are reflected here. The examples and comments are grouped according to types of acute service.

Accident and emergency care

Accident and emergency (A & E) departments are affected by the area in which they are situated. One such department in District C had no specific recruitment problems as they were able to employ new staff completing the in-house training course. However, the Sister here emphasised the importance of having experienced staff. One of the biggest problems was maternity leave, and replacing such staff is complicated by a management decision not to take on *temporary* staff. This decision seemed to defy logic, as a Staff Nurse in the department had been 'acting up' for two years.

A suggestion that staff should *job-share* was turned down, but some young Sisters who were pregnant were planning to request that this decision be reconsidered, as the shift system lent itself to job sharing. This A & E department had to close for a week owing to staff shortages. It seemed irrational that young doctors spend six months working in A & E, usually learning on the job, backed up by senior staff, but for nurses such short-term appointments seem to be unacceptable. The blockage of efforts to recruit temporary or part-time staff seems to be an example of *inflexible nurse managers clinging to principles that go unchallenged*, resulting in a loss of experienced people once they have children, or a lost opportunity to train up temporary staff who could act as stop-gaps in the future. Furthermore, this was happening within a district that was promoting flexibility.

This A & E department had 40 whole-time equivalents (WTEs) and saw, on average, 1000 patients each week. The number was increasing annually. Although ECGs were performed by technicians working 40 hours per week, nurses were also spending 120 hours a week doing ECGs, each one taking around 15 minutes. In addition, a whole day could be spent on the telephone finding beds when there are acute shortages, some patients could wait for admission on hard trolleys for up to seven hours.

In the admissions area, there could be 30 incoming calls in an hour from patients and doctors wanting advice; only an experienced nurse can cope adequately with these enquiries. *The incidence of major trauma and death in the department leads to a high level of stress.* Nurses have to deal with relatives who are suddenly bereaved, and also support themselves and junior medical staff. Nurses need training and experience in coping with the effects of these experiences both on themselves and on their colleagues.

A Sister in another A & E department said that very busy times often resulted in patients and staff becoming short-tempered. Complaints about waiting times caused nurses to feel a sense of failure, and resentment that public expectations were too high. The sheer pressure of work left little or no time for talking to patients and they consequently felt neglected, and complained. On one occasion, there was only one trained member of staff on duty who had to stay on 13 hours in order to cover the department.

These comments raise questions about attitudes of the public towards service providers, and the attitudes of nurses and doctors to patients, which are coloured by the pressure and upsetting nature of much of the work. Either way, there is a need to educate the professionals more effectively in dealing with the public, and conversely, taking steps to improve public understanding of the way A & E departments function.

The nursing division of North West Thames RHA has issued guidelines on dealing with stress among nurses and for coping with bereavements, in order to help nurses to work in environments where there are high levels of stress and high death rates, such as in A & E departments.

Surgical care

A Sister on a busy surgical ward reported:

> Health care is now more care of the elderly in both medicine and surgery. There is a feeling that we are in a 'business', and the general lack of money impinges on us all the time. There is a production-line feeling, which is having a qualitative effect on morale. Nurses, in order to be motivated, must feel 'good' about their work because they have so many unpleasant things to do. If, at the end of the day, they are giving less than their best, if for example they have no time to hold the hand of a dying patient, as happens now, then they feel demoralized.

In fact, in this case, this Sister's ward was fully staffed, and she had a stable workforce who had not changed in 18 months. It could be asked then, what was happening here that created a feeling of high pressure? In this particular hospital, there had been a massive reduction in beds partly because of overspending, and partly because of consistent underusage. This had led to a situation that was echoed by other staff throughout the same hospital of continual bed shortages.

Sisters at this hospital complained that the telephone constantly rung with requests for empty beds for patients to be admitted. Negotiating discharges or transfers of patients was a continuous pressure as this Sister explains:

> Patients are bed-fodder, there is no time to care. When a patient died recently I wanted to leave the bed empty for a while, all the other patients knew and were upset. But there was a patient waiting elsewhere in the hospital and the bed had to be filled immediately. There are now few low-dependency patients, the slightest sign of being able to cope and they are told they can go home, often before stitches are removed.
>
> Patients and staff come before doctors. In the old days we did ward rounds with the consultants but this is delegated to other staff now, as there is no time to be part of an entourage as in the

past. Now I have seven consultants on a 22-bed ward, and they all come at different times. However, the medical staff have been very supportive and have drawn to the attention of management the bed shortages and pressures this creates, this makes us feel less isolated.

This whole testimony is imbued with a sense of continual crisis, this Sister had long experience (17 years at that level), and had also worked in Africa. She was in a position to assess the difference in the NHS in the past, and the effect on nurses now. This Sister had difficulty in adjusting to some aspects of the new management outlook. For example, delegation of responsibility to junior staff on ward rounds was part of a philosophy toward greater continuity of care. She emphasised that she spent a good deal of time on 'keeping staff happy so they stay', and 'being the leader but making changes together'. Commenting on management she had this to say:

There are too many non-clinical people running the hospital at the moment – it is becoming depersonalised, we are no longer individuals, people are classified. Staff are categorised, patients are labelled 'waiting list' or 'emergency', managers always telephone or send memos, they are not recognisable to staff. Nurses who are managers always come to the ward. They realise that, in this job, personal contact is important. Nevertheless, they are becoming more and more desk-bound. I feel I could resolve many problems myself that I take to my manager if I had the responsibility and could take more decisions personally.

I now have to act in the middle-manager role, and know how difficult it is. I have to be on call for the whole hospital and finding staff is not easy, and finding empty beds. There is much more financial involvement of middle managers, so the job has become more complicated.

Privatisation of cleaning services meant that the domestic worker was no longer part of a team, and is another example of the depersonalising process that is happening. We are all overstretched, and therefore being a team is important in order to support and protect each other.

This interview identifies some of the main issues that recur with great frequency in other clinical settings. The *higher throughputs*, *the reduction in beds, the gap between nursing ideals and the realities of ward life, the higher dependencies of patients and the corresponding increase in hard, physical labour that is involved with heavy, intensive nursing, the changing management structure, and depersonalisation of many aspects of that transformation, the continual atmosphere of crisis.*

On the positive side, this Sister has managed to maintain a stable and committed workforce in a situation where extra pairs of hands are scarce, learner numbers fluctuate and where there is little control over admissions, even in situations where the ward is full of high-dependency patients. To some extent this reflected the holistic nurse management system of District C. However, the emphasis on support for ward nursing staff and setting aside time for this aspect was an important factor in retaining their commitment. It should be added here that there was little complaint about administrative load, as the same ward clerk had been on the ward for 15 years, which was also very unusual but she undertook a major part of the administrative work.

Contrast this interview with a young Charge Nurse's views in a London teaching hospital in District D. He was appointed four years after qualification to a general surgical ward. The ward was also fully staffed to establishment levels; however, a recent pilot study for Excelcare System revealed that a revision of staffing levels was needed, and that they were actually functioning at minimum levels. The workforce, on the whole, was composed of newly-qualified Staff Nurses and they had been unable to recruit an experienced Senior Staff Nurse for six months.

It has to be acknowledged that, in this hospital, most of the care is done by people under 25 years of age, and that includes many of the junior medical staff as well. The workload has increased, the types of dependencies have changed – we no longer have long-term surgical patients but higher throughputs, also shift patterns have changed thus reducing overlaps so there is still no less work. We always *feel* as though we are working at minimal staff levels.

We do not have regular staff meetings – they are only random and are usually cathartic sessions to purge bad feelings that build up. These outbursts are usually related to quality of work, and a falling short of ideals, not just as individuals, but as a group.

The problem is that nurses expect strong leadership because of the way they have been educated. Work is very formalised and the structure emphasises discipline, and there is consequently a reluctance by individual nurses to err from the norm. By anticipating an authoritarian structure, they also expect punishment for deviations. Recently, a junior nurse who made a drug error expected retribution and cried, in spite of the fact I just talked to her about drug policy 'in general' to avoid a recurrence of the mistake. Really, the emphasis in the past on discipline, authority and punishment leads ultimately to a lack of independent judgement by nurses. Learning in the clinical area is an educational process not a system of repression.

Personally, I feel stressed by some situations on the ward, but feel I must learn to cope because I want to climb the ladder to a higher level job. One of the most stressful things is poor ward hygiene – I feel I have no control over this, and I go through the 'usual channels' and get nowhere. Poor food, unreliable transport for patients, the rudeness of doctors to staff, and the unsupportive attitudes of nurses towards each other, are also dimensions of stress.

I am not happy with the way things are. *I am not 'the manager' of my ward, but merely the supervisor*. I have only partial control over my environment, and cannot change most things. We are supposed to work alongside other services, but it's not like that. We meet them all as nurses, we dress up their sometimes inadequate provision and try to make it all right for the patient, because *in spite of everything they think that we are personally responsible for the service they receive*.

In the post-Griffiths period there has been no visible change at this level, but there is worry about the new structures, as above the ward there won't be anyone necessarily called 'a nurse'. Junior Sisters particularly need the security of the knowledge that they have an experienced nurse at a higher level. Since the Griffiths changes, however, relationships have decreased with higher managers, we feel forgotten and neglected here. *I have only had one appraisal, and because of the high turnover of my staff I have performed no appraisals, only exit interviews*.

I need to see the leader of nursing, the knowledge that there is one is not enough, not any more. They hardly come at all. You need to feel valued by your employers and your colleagues. This makes me feel that I want to leave nursing sometimes. Feeling undervalued by managers, is reinforced by attitudes of doctors and even patients as they don't seem to understand the constraints we work under.

This ward is a popular ward, there is a queue of students for jobs here. But with higher pressures to push patients out, more complicated surgery, and complex treatments for terminal conditions, greater skill and patience is required of the nurse to meet individual needs of patients, and it requires an increasing amount of effort to do the same job. Most of our Staff Nurses only stay six to nine months.

A third Sister in another hospital in District D was trying to do a Diploma in Management, but the increasing pressure of work was making this difficult to maintain, and she explained why as follows:

I go off for this course 1 day a week, I am finding it tiring because the job is so busy. Most of the people on the course are not in nursing – so I see things from a different angle. But it is so tiring beause my job is so busy. I have to have a day in mid-week for the course, on the other days, which are 'operating days', the ward is very busy. In addition, I have to have the bleep from the middle manager to cover her patch. I know this is to give me higher management experience but it is too much, and is a nonsense when I am so busy.

Sisters feel, in this situation, that they are being exploited and treated badly, and not being developed. I feel a sense of failure if I have to say I really cannot do things. My manager asks, 'Why not?', and I have to explain that I have eight patients back from theatre and cannot answer telephone requests. It's difficult, as they say it doesn't look good if I give the bleep back to them, and I feel I cannot make progress because my job has so many critical practical demands.

Last Monday was particularly chaotic, two trained staff were off sick, I had to go to Court about an industrial compensation claim from a nurse who had hurt her back lifting a patient, I could not go to my study day, and I had hardly any sleep because of a disturbance at home.

My middle manager was kind and supportive, *but overall my*

continual absences from the ward because of the management course
and the bleep-carrying have a detrimental effect on my staff. You
need time to develop and motivate staff, or they leave and
find jobs outside the NHS. My priority must be to support my
staff and quite often they are literally terrified by what they are
expected to do. I have had no ward clerk for nine months.
Every day there are petty problems like blood pressure
machines out of order and I don't have the power to see that
they are mended quickly, as the Assistant DNS is the budget
holder. I've tried to get a commode with wheels for two years,
I ordered a fan recently – nothing has happened; it took six
months and four requisitions to get two notice boards ...
sometimes I feel that administration/management 'is as useful
as a chocolate fireguard'.

Four months ago, I told administation we needed new
equipment: there was no response. It is all very frustrating, and
a blight to my own morale and ward staff. Management seems
remote to nurses, those at higher levels are not visible very often.
It would be nice to have some praise at the end of the week. Pay
is not everything, being valued, having status at this level and
recognition is just as important.

A Sister in another hospital in District D said that changing her
ward to a high-dependency ward with an establishment set from a
Telford Study performed four years before caused 'fearful pressure'.
She explained:

Six Staff Nurses left all at once, we did not understand what was
happening. I felt worried all the time and inadequate and no
longer up to the job. It made me cold and angry towards people.
I couldn't say 'no' to people and more and more work piled up
on staff and *I felt that saying 'no' showed a personal failing.*

I did an 'assertion course' and learnt to say 'no' to doctors. I
had to find my own feet before supporting others. The problem
was that there was an acute need for extra staff, and there
seemed to be no mechanism to get help.

My middle manager comes twice a week, memos are given
about off-duty and we discuss the odd problem and that's just
about it. Some months ago when faced with an acute staff
shortage I went 'circuitously' to the top of the hierarchy to

complain, it was the only way. Last year I had to *demand* an appraisal, as I have had no feedback. This new middle-management structure is really no different to the old one, it is 'a rose by another name', at least that's how it feels. *Actually I could do with more autonomy in some respects.*

Yet another Sister in the same hospital in the neurosurgery department complained:

I am constantly berated for overspending but no one will tell me what the budget is. The manager is now less visible on the wards, and staff feel more remote. He is more burdened with administration when, before, a daily ward round was made. It is a great loss here. Five beds have been closed for 12 months because of low staffing levels, sometimes I have to leave junior members of staff (third-year students) in charge of the ward, our staff are very inexperienced and cannot do drug rounds, observations or IV infusions. In these circumstances, consultants are more selective about admissions as the situation is potentially dangerous.

I fill in, on a daily basis, the patient's dependencies *but never see the results,* there is no outcome and no relationship with staffing levels so far as I can see. I often work an extra couple of hours to keep things going. I wanted to do a management course, but if you are working your backside off 24 hours of the day it's too much. I felt upset that I couldn't do it.

These interviews highlight many of the problems faced by Sisters/ Charge Nurses in the surgical clinical area: high throughputs, more distant, unresponsive and overloaded middle management, clumsy systems for ordering and maintaining equipment, frustration with inadequate cleaning services, increasing pressure to take on wider responsibilities, lack of time to develop their own careers, lack of appraisal systems, or reciprocal communications from higher management about important requests, and an overwhelming sense of feeling undervalued, and of failing the patient and not living up to professional and public expectations. Unfortunately, these expressions of feeling were far more frequently and cogently expressed than the positive ones, and therefore require greater emphasis here.

Medical care

A young Sister in an inner London hospital remarked:

> Not a single member of my staff wants to be a Ward Sister. I
> want to be a counsellor for nurses to help staff to cope with
> dying patients and relatives and cut down on the staff turnover
> in nursing. *You see, most of the people at the moment giving direct
> care in nursing here are under 21 years of age. Only the consultant
> and registrar and myself are over 25 years.* Their ideas about
> nursing are often too theoretical, when the clinical direct care
> role is often mismatched.
>
> I am fed up about patients dying in dirty rooms – I find it bad
> enough dealing with young people dying but being powerless to
> make any improvement in the environment makes things worse.
> The support services have not improved since the new
> management.
>
> I can't stand having the bleep, it is an *extra burden* and takes
> me away from the ward so much. I have had five SNMs since
> I started here two years ago. I've had one appraisal in the
> whole time. When the patients write nice things I put it in a
> scrap book, so all the staff can see and feel encouraged. The
> doctors here are also very supportive and praise our work, but
> we do not have it from nurse managers.
>
> Keeping standards up is important, nurses want to come and
> work here and are enthusiastic, I must have time to respond and
> be interested, it is a chicken and egg situation . . .

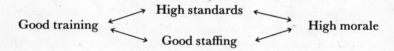

> The problem is that I have 25 staff in all, including the learners,
> and arranging off-duty, orientations, training learners and so
> on, all has to be done in addition to the central business of
> looking after the patient. With such a large group it is difficult to
> maintain personal contact with everyone.
>
> *The middle managers are not seen now, their jobs have changed
> and they have no time to come here.* I try not to think of
> everyday crises as pressures or stress, as nurse managers do,

but positively as 'new challenges' that must be overcome. But we do need managers who are nurses who can argue about the viability of admitting some patients who need complex nursing and who are undergoing risky procedures. Nurse managers can argue for planned admissions more confidently with a consultant as they would be more aware of all the issues involved and of the training specifications of the ward.

Another problem outlined by a Charge Nurse was the lack of further training for middle managers:

> They are creating new jobs, but putting the old SNMs in them without further training. Formerly, it was a very autocratic type of management, this does not work. I don't believe in it, we are all on first-name terms in the ward, this does not lessen respect for my authority. My greater experience and knowledge gain respect. *There is no appraisal system here, no pat on the back and too much negative feedback. We never see the UGM on the wards and no one knows the senior management or who they are.*

Constant instabilities at ward level are a further problem. At one London teaching hospital, a Sister explains the practical problems in ward and staff management that this poses:

> Here, there is almost 100 per cent turnover of staff every year. I do appraisals, not to be critical, but to help staff perform better. But it doesn't make them want to stay longer, just occasionally a Staff Nurse will stay for a year. The atmosphere is never stable, people tend to come and go in groups. I'm just getting 'things to jell', and they leave, and only the most junior staff remain. Sometimes this means we definitely have the wrong mixture, but this is how things are and I have to accept it.

The back-up system from the middle-management tier was also extremely unstable in one hospital. *One Sister complained that she had nine SNMs in four years and had never had an appraisal.* Responsibility for staffing the hospital and trouble-shooting had been pushed so low that *often very inexperienced Sisters were on duty*, and that those most willing to carry out these duties were not necessarily those best suited to do so.

Teaching on the wards also creates conflicts between the ideal and the real and possible. *Some Sisters feel that, in practice, the nursing model excludes the medical model too much.* For example, one Sister explains:

> The ENB prefer the nursing model, that is to say, you don't write, 'nursing care of the patient following myocardial infarction' on the work sheet but, 'the nurse's responsibilities towards health education with particular reference to patients following a heart attack, his present and future needs'. A straightforward lesson on the renal or cardiac system is frowned upon by the hierarchy, but I think nurses have to understand doctors' terms as they work so closely together. In order to understand the effects of renal failure you have to know what it is, I think.
>
> The urge towards greater independence of the patient is a model that forgets how dependent a patient needs to be, at least, for a period. In an acute medical ward, 'self-care' is out of place in some instances, and nursing models are sometimes too complex for the average nurse to sort out objectives in relation to the patient's condition, and the reasons for doing things.

Dealing with death in some of the specialist medical facilities was also a major stress in some Ward Sisters' roles. In renal units, bone marrow transplant or cancer treatment cases, death is more common and more often involves younger patients. One Sister on a renal unit describes the environment:

> We had ten deaths in a very short period just before Christmas, staff morale was at rock bottom. The workload was so high that everyone was always going home late, and never felt that they had finished. They needed to express their feelings: we now have a nurse counsellor once a week, a group meeting at least every two months. This helps me be a better manager because it creates understanding at different levels. This is why you need a senior manager who is not just a booking agency, not inundated with secretarial work, but someone who can be involved and really understand the issues. We need continuity in back-up as there is a high dependency on agency staff, and high turnovers, and we are constantly striving to provide a consistent standard of care for patients in the face of all this instability.

At another hospital, failure of SN management to give adequate back-up was keenly felt when a mortuary attendant refused to allow a patient's wife access to her husband for five hours. The Sister took this up with senior management, and old guidelines were uncovered that had not been circulated. The mortuary attendant was persistently rude and unhelpful, and the Sister felt that little had changed even after this incident. The failure to circulate procedures about access to patients who have died, and the obstructiveness of those responsible made this Sister's job more difficult. A sense of frustration about the inhumanity of the system was not helped by weak middle-management action.

On some occasions, the Sisters' own inability to sort out their own problems is evident. Complaints about being 'stale' with work and lack of interest by middle managers could be countered by criticisms of lack of Sisters' initiative to go out and update themselves. *It seems too often that Sisters/Charge Nurses are waiting for guidance from above, and not using their own motivation for self improvement.*

On the medical wards, the main areas of concern were as follows:

1 extra duties for higher management on-call for the hospital;
2 lack of appraisal or positive feedback from middle-management to wards;
3 rapid turnover of staff leaving the most junior staff to provide continuity;
4 the gap in teaching between theory and practice;
5 the complexity of some of nursing care models;
6 the inexperience of some Sisters doing on-call hospital duties;
7 the impact on staff and relatives of death, and humanizing the system for everyone; and
8 the expectation that motivation must come from 'above' more than the self.

Intensive care

Intensive care units (ITUs) are the technologically advanced nursing areas, and are the dramatic background to many fundamental dilemmas in nursing today. The battle for life is fought daily, the medical model is dominant and in conflict from time to time with nursing models, as one Sister described it succinctly – 'It's glitzy medicine'.

In this environment, the limits of medicine are reached, and in some cases are 'pushed further than we ought to go', according to one Sister. In the high-profile environment of the teaching hospital, the workforce is stable, sickness rates are low, burn-out minimal and hierarchy muted and relaxed.

> Here it is not just a question of more pay – that's just the surface
> of the problem, *it's social value really*. Society does not value us,
> if I go to a party and tell someone what I do, I can see how
> boring they think I am, people don't value nurses. Really at
> work I am like a director in the middle of the room conducting a
> drama, without me the whole structure would fall apart.

This Sister taught on the course at the ITU, liaised with medical staff, taught junior medical staff about the machinery, and counselled staff and relatives. She emphasised the importance of the last function:

> It's not learnt by osmosis, as some people seem to think, we
> need to be trained to help others. We are, more than ever, the
> patient's advocate as they are usually unconscious, and cannot
> stand up for their rights – particularly where pain is concerned.
> Giving the right amount of analgesic causes conflict. I feel I
> could scream sometimes as some medical staff are concentrating
> more on throughputs and economic and scientific priorities. For
> this reason, *nurses need to keep their influence in general management,
> to maintain a clinical impact at that level and maintain a humanistic
> perspective rather than a scientific or economic view.*

On these ITUs, the usual problems of lack of clerical support and poor standards of cleaning services arise. An example of the frustrations was as follows:

> At 11 o'clock the cleaner disappeared, she'd gone off sick and
> didn't tell anyone. Since *privatization we have lost our regular
> cleaner who had been with us eight years. She was not daunted
> by all the equipment; now they have no training and we have no
> control. It's not cost-effective because of all the hassle, the 'phone*

calls, the dirty environment – all this can't be costed.

The pay for the cleaners and people like the technicians is too low; and yet we need their skills, it's very important to have close relationships with all staff, everyone is important here. I've been asking for some clerical help for three years, I would be willing to lose a Staff Nurse if it would be possible.

We are highly dependent here on agency nurses, often *our own staff* are working agency because managers say that it's cheaper than working overtime. The agency down the road has grown colossally over the last three years and now has huge offices. It makes you think that it would be better to have our own bank.

In this particular hospital continuous changes in the management structure were felt to be very unsettling:

It's tearing the hospital apart, and personally I'm losing faith and feel I want to leave. It's a pity really as I had thought that the Griffiths Report was a positive thing.

In both these testimonies, the importance of supportive and consistent middle management was emphasised. One ITU had a more stable environment than the other because it had a pool of recruits from the in-house training course. Without this source, the supply was largely dependent on supplements from the agency. *Ironically, the same staff were employed through the external private agency in order to save the NHS overtime payments, it could lead to abuse, pushing staff to work over-long hours.*

In this unstable environment, the higher management was also marked by change and instability, which had a 'domino' effect at ward level. The close relationships between medical and nursing staff were also characteristic of these areas: conflicts arose over the methods and objectives of sustaining life or maintaining its quality. To argue the case, nurses needed a confident and articulate higher-management structure which was clinically well-informed.

Needing to feel valued, again, was a theme either intrinsic to the interview responses, or openly expressed. The intense involvement with patients having bone-marrow transplants, traumatic accidents, suicides, overdoses of drugs and alcohol, major surgery or medical crises, created an atmosphere of constant high drama, which nurses felt it was hard to convey to outsiders. These complex problems not only demanded high levels of technical expertise, but also enormous emotional and psychological input in terms of sustaining relatives, and acting as patient's advocate.

Nursing in the ITU is a magnification of nursing in the acute hospital; the nurse is the primary carer, the technical expert, the mediator between medical staff, management, relatives and patients. These tasks require a wide spectrum of training, and a stable support structure to enable this to function well.

Comment

Managers are fond of saying that our greatest assets are people, but these assets are *usually accounted for as costs rather than capital that needs to be invested in.* To give people greater responsibility and job achievement means they need continuous information on performance against standards. This is lacking at the ward level in many areas of the Health Service.

The problem is that too much involvement with 'functions' such as staffing the wards leaves too little time to address what Drucker (1979) calls the *'conscience' functions of higher management,* that is to say, the 'support' work that enables workers to achieve and feel valued. Those in the new middle-management roles, all too often, are unable to carry out the necessary 'conscience' functions for nurses.

Summary

1   The personal testimony of some Sisters/Charge Nurses identified any common problems. Inflexible managers unwilling to recruit part-timers or temporary help were a source of frustration to some Sisters.

2   Higher workloads were often associated with higher throughputs. The business management philosophy was felt by some to depersonalise aspects of nursing. Comforting patients or dealing with death were marginalised by the institutional needs of providing maximum use of beds. This created a conflict between nursing philosophy of holistic and individual care, and the organisational need to rationalise resources.

3   The larger workload of middle managers had transformed their image into that of 'pen pushers'. Their lack of clinical contact was frequently commented on together with the feeling that many middle managers had become remote. The increasing administrative load described in Chapter 8 may explain the change, but it was interpreted at ward level as a sign that management did not care, and had become depersonalised.

4   This conception was reinforced by a lack of systematic appraisal, or positive reinforcement from middle managers. The rapid turnover at these levels made it difficult to build consistent relationships over a long period between Sisters and middle managers. This may explain why some feel isolated and undervalued by the organisation and why a remote image of management was perceived by those at ward level.

5   Continuing stress was another aspect of the Ward Sister's role. There have been attempts to respond. There are regional guidelines, and in some areas counselling services for staff. Nevertheless, the youthfulness and lack of training and experience of many staff make this an important area for middle managers to give support, both directly and by influencing admission rates.

6   Personal development is an area where many Ward Sisters expect guidance from higher management. Some were very passive about further training and did not actively seek their own development, but looked to senior managers for advice. There seemed few structured opportunities to gain wider experience other than short courses. By comparison, the junior medical staff had a more varied and ordered career path at this point.

7   A sense of not being valued by society was another frustration. This was coupled with a real feeling that sometimes the public did not understand the nature of nursing or the pressures caused by lack of nurses, cleaners or clerical staff. Nurses were the visible human face of the NHS, and possibly for this reason were often blamed for its inadequacies. They consequently had a higher sense of failure than other occupational groups, as they were in direct daily contact with the public more than most other health professionals.

8   Nurses often acted as agency replacements for their own unit to save the organisation money. They showed a high sense of

commitment to the service and to the patient. This meant
working extra hours to help out in times of extreme shortage
but probably contributed to high rates of burn-out and absence.

9   Sisters/Charge Nurses saw themselves as patients' advocates.
On some occasions, this meant conflicting with medical personnel. This led to tensions in areas where clinicians were not
prepared to listen, or who were openly rude or dismissive of
nurses' opinions.

10 In general, the Ward Sister/Charge Nurse is at the most
conflict-laden point in the whole health care system, as she or
he is the person who coordinates other services, takes the strain
off other professionals from cleaners to doctors while, at the
same time, having little actual control over the arena in which
she or he works. Middle management has become more remote,
bureaucratic and overloaded.

11
Conclusions

———————— ◆ ————————

Conclusion 1

The internal reorganisation of the NHS set off by the Griffiths Report is one of the most important to have taken place since it began. It has affected every level in the Service from the Department of Health right down to ward and community level.

Conclusion 2

Its two central principles involved maximum delegation of authority to act downwards in the organisation and the reduction of separate parallel lines of management for each occupational group. Line management responsibilities were to be concentrated so far as possible in one general manager at each level of the Service.

Conclusion 3

Nursing was the largest separately managed workforce in the Service. It was therefore importantly affected by these proposed changes.

Conclusion 4

As the authority to restructure units and districts had been devolved, the extent of change varied widely within the region studied here (North West Thames). Similar reorganisations have taken place in other parts of the country.

Conclusion 5

Major changes in the responsibility for nursing staff have occurred at senior management levels, at district and also unit level. There has been an attempt to delegate more responsibility to the Ward Sisters/ Charge Nurses in the ward or community. All these changes in posts, personnel and job content occurred at a time when nursing was under strain (see Chapters 2 & 3).

Conclusion 6

Griffiths reported at precisely the point in the Health Service's history when demographic demands were growing and real resources allocated to it ceased to grow (see Table 1.1). Fundamental changes in society, and advances in medical science increased expectations and changed attitudes towards death. The demands of an ageing population were also putting a strain on the Service. This had a cascade effect on nurses and others in the front line who had to absorb the effects of highly dependent people receiving more treatments. This made the job of nursing increasingly stressful at the time when the pool of young people on which it relied was declining (see Chapters 2 & 3).

Conclusion 7

At the same time, there were unresolved and deep-seated conflicts within nursing between union and professional values, about the nature of education and training, about the structure of the profession and issues of power within the Health Service. In addition, there has been considerable industrial unrest, related to pay and value in society (see Chapters 2, 3 & 4).

Conclusion 8

All of these factors combined put young nurses and Sisters/Charge Nurses on the wards and in the community in a very difficult and stressful situation. Many Ward Sisters/Charge Nurses in the acute hospitals that we interviewed had been in post for no longer than two years. The continued stability of the nursing service required firm, confident and capable leadership at every level. Yet it was at precisely this time that the Griffiths restructuring began.

Whatever its long-term advantages, the short-term effect was to disrupt nursing leadership and support. There was a period of professional uncertainty at the top as nurses had to adjust to a new concept of management. In some instances, line management became separated from professional leadership. New rules and relationships had to be learned. The traditional hierarchical nature of nursing meant it was less well-adapted to respond to these new pressures.

One District General Manager who had put nursing on top of his agenda appointed a Director of Nurse Education in combination with a District Nursing Adviser. She was given resources and freedom to act, and had produced a significant impact on nursing recruitment, retention and morale, and reduced budget overspending on manpower. Each district faced different problems and no general prescription for this level of responsibility is possible, but the conception of the DNA role in this district provides an excellent model (see Chapter 6).

Conclusion 9

Most unit structures were being reorganised to eliminate separate lines of nursing management. In the new style, units were being divided into sub-units. In acute hospitals, these sub-units were based on the constituent services such as inpatient services, theatres and accident and emergency services. In the community units, the new patterns differed. Usually they were divided on a location basis or, in others, on a client group basis.

Conclusion 10

The split between professional leadership and accountability and the mainline daily management of the nursing workforce could produce problems, sometimes serious. General managers sought to minimise the effect by appointing nurses to head those sub-units that employed most nurses in the acute hospital sector and in the community services. Professional accountability was to a head of nursing within each unit. In fact, this meant that nurses were moving into widened general management positions on a large scale. Our interviews suggested that the individuals concerned were enjoying their increased responsibilities, although there were stresses caused by over-extended responsibilities and more administrative work.

Conclusion 11

The most problematic level of work in nursing, as in other welfare bureaucracies, is level three, that is the organisation of work over a range of settings and situations. Radical reductions in middle management to meet financial goals placed greater workloads on those at this level. Most middle managers appointed were nurses who had add-on responsibilities for a specific area of service. However, although titles of jobs changed from Senior Nurse Manager (SNM) to Service Manager (SM) or Location Manager, power relationships based on traditional patterns between doctors and nurses and their occupational groups did not necessarily change with restructuring arrangements. In the acute hospitals, middle managers were responsible for more wards and, in some instances, well over a hundred staff. Most of their time was spent on crisis management, ensuring there were enough staff on the wards. This was a largely administrative task, and a substantial part could have been delegated to a non-nurse administrative assistant.

Conclusion 12

Where nurse managers at this level had been given extended roles as SM, they had responsibility, in theory, for a workforce that included other personnel as well as nurses. However, in reality, this had not matched formal responsibilities as they had not been given budget-holding powers and other staff were not, in practice, accountable to them. Doctors did not readily accept nurses in middle-management roles, and in some cases refused to acknowledge them. Nor did those we interviewed believe they had had appropriate, or indeed in most cases any, training for their extended roles. Shift systems made access to training more difficult than for those in regular administrative posts with office hours.

Conclusion 13

In contrast, the nature of the work of Ward Sisters/Charge Nurses had changed little, although the pressures and strains had increased. They perceived the middle managers as mere 'pen-pushers' in many cases, or thought that they were too overburdened with routine functional tasks. Most of the issues they discussed together were shortages in staffing. They also felt, in many cases, that they received little positive support or praise, as middle managers were too busy staffing wards daily. Two-thirds of Sisters/Charge Nurses complained of increasing workloads. Commitment to the job was nevertheless high, and only 4 per cent said that they wanted to leave the NHS. However, most wanted more control over all the staff on the ward and budgets. They complained that their nursing establishments were set by tradition and were not systematically and regularly reappraised. There were a few examples of this happening, and it had positive results, as it had a stabilising effect on the workforce.

Conclusion 14

An analysis of nursing history (Chapters 2 & 3) has shown that nurses have, since the nineteenth century, consistently adapted to changing social and medical needs. In this reorganisation, the profession has had to make major adjustments to its managerial style and concepts of nursing. On balance, nurses are now well established at middle-management level and will be in an excellent position to be the general managers of the future, having both expert knowledge and enhanced management skills. Changes in nurse education and in attitudes towards women in the Health Service will also provide greater opportunities for nurses as leaders in the NHS of the future.

Appendix

————————— ◆ —————————

Methodology

The purpose of the research project was to observe and comment on the changing structure of the management of nursing in the post-Griffiths period. The principal methodology used was the anthropological method of observation and interviews with key Health Service personnel. This method has the value of giving an in-depth understanding of the infrastructure of organisations, and can illuminate areas that are not revealed by mass-survey techniques. It enables us to understand organisations from the point of view of those who work in them.

The project began in October 1985, at a time when all the districts in the North West Thames region had newly appointed District General Managers. However, it was not until April 1986 that all the Unit General Managers were in post. This affected the outcome of the first six-month period of research field work, as most unit structures were not fully completed, and the research was conducted in an environment of change and uncertainty.

With these factors in mind, a structured interview was devised to encompass a wide range of topics, in an effort to incorporate both structural factors and the views of Senior Nurse Managers. The interview was taped and a written copy sent to each interviewee for comments, or amendments, to validate the material. Over the fieldwork period, 78 SNMs, (CNOs, DNSs, and some nurses in Planning and Personnel were interviewed), and a small number of SNOs and a Personnel Officer in the 14 districts. Interviews lasted, on average, about two hours, which gave ample time for self expression, and in-depth reflection. The report published in the first year, focused on particular issues that dominated the discussions, and the results were a collation of interview material published in the report *The Nursing Management Function after Griffiths* (Glennerster & Owens, 1986).

Further informal and unstructured interviews were conducted with senior nurses at regional level and, in addition, staff from Personnel, the Treasurer's Department, as well as the RGM, RNO and the RMO. To collect the DGM and UGM point of view, short interviews were undertaken with all 14 DGMs and with 18 UGMs selected from seven districts. The selection of the districts was based on a variety of criteria as follows:

1 a nurse had been appointed as a general manager;
2 where a CNO was retained, but has a hybrid role incorporating other functions, for example that of Quality Assurance Officer, Nurse Adviser or Head of Nurse Education;
3 a nurse was a mini-manager or Assistant General Manager (for example, a head of hospital or a Location Community manager);
4 a DNS was acting as a Nurse Adviser and retains operational management control; or
5 where a district had retained many features of an earlier pattern of organisation.

The overall approach focused on the *structural* elements of organisational change and its effect on nurse management. However, personal points of view are used to illustrate the effects on individuals. Case studies are also used to give a human face to organisational issues, and to place abstract and critical discussion in some tangible context. The overall aim of the methodology used in the first year was to give a sense of the problems and issues that faced individual general managers and nurses against the wider canvas of the social and structural constraints within the organisation of the NHS in the North West Thames region.

In the second year, the researchers focused on four districts from the region. These districts were chosen because they represented different environments for the delivery of health care, for example, an inner-city district, a rural one and two from peripheral London locations. In addition, the DNAs had different hybrid roles. The research did not concentrate on particular district problems but more on the common problems that assail nurse management regardless of location. The methodology used was largely observation at meetings. These meetings were between nurses and managers at district and unit level. Many meetings attended were individual exchanges between different levels of staff, or alternatively, larger group meetings including DHAs, DMBs, UMBs, DNACs, and meetings of Sisters or SNOs, or clinical practice groups, totalling over 150 meetings. Information was supplemented by personal interviews, and follow-up interviews with key staff. The content of meetings was recorded, and the principal subject matter classified and computerised, to give a firmer idea of major areas of discussion.

The main basis of the methodology was network analysis, tracing how different managers related to nursing. Some maps of these communication networks and case studies illustrated the functioning of the system of nurse management in the district context. The results were summarised in a second interim report (Glennerster & Owens, 1987).

In addition, informal interviews with staff at regional level, with DGMs and other personnel such as Treasurers, as well as a variety of managers of services and with high levels of nursing staff, also supplemented the network analysis. In the final year of research, structured interviews of middle managers and Charge Nurses/Ward Sisters in nine acute hospitals explored the content of those roles in the new structures. In total, 92 interviews were undertaken, and 85 analysed by classifying the contents using an SPSSX programme. This gave some idea of the substance of the communications between levels of management.

Over the whole study period, there were nearly 400 interviews and meetings attended by the researchers. The size and complexity of the fieldwork area meant that it was impossible to incorporate all the available data. We have chosen to concentrate on the main structural changes in organisational form, and on the processes of management of nursing services in the context of the Health Service as a whole.

Bibliography

———— ◆ ————

Aaron, H. J. & Schwartz, W. B. (1984) *The Painful Prescription*, The Brooking Institute, Washington DC.

Abel-Smith, B. (1960) *A History of the Nursing Profession*, Heinemann, London.

Abel-Smith, B. (1964) *The Hospitals 1800–1948*, Heinemann, London.

Abel-Smith, B. (1984a) 'Assessing the balance sheet', in *The Future of the Welfare State*, ed. H. Glennerster, Heinemann, London.

Abel-Smith, B. (1984b) *Cost Containment in Health Care*, Occasional Papers in Social Administration, No. 73, Bedford Press, London.

Adams, J. R. (1969) 'From association to union: professional organisation of asylum attendants 1869–1919', *Brit. J. Soc.*, **20**.

Anderson, F. (1987) Doctors despair of management, *HSJ*, **97**, 9.7.87.

Ariès, P. (1976) *Western Attitudes to Death from the Middle Ages to the Present*, Boyers, London.

Armstrong, M. (1981) *Practical Nurse Management*, Arnold, London.

Atkinson, P. (1983) The reproduction of the professional community, in *The Sociology of the Professions*, ed. R. Dingwall and P. Lewis, Macmillan, London.

Baly, M. E. (1973) *Nursing and Social Change*, Heinemann, London.

Banks, G. T. (1979) 'Programme budgeting for DHSS', in *Planning for Welfare*, Blackwells, Oxford.

Bassett, P. (1988) 'The professionals who refuse to put patients at risk'. *Financial Times*, 22 January.

Bealing, M. (1986) 'Some are more equal than others', *HSSJ*, **96**, 30.1.86.

Beatham, D. (1987) *Bureaucracy*, Open University Press, Milton Keynes.

Becker, H. S., Geer, B., Hughes, E. L. & Strauss, A. L. (1960) *The Boys in White: Student Culture in Medical School*, University of Chicago Press, Chicago.

Beer, S. (1982) *Modern British Politics: A Study of Parties and Pressure Groups*, Faber, London.

Bellaby, P. & Oribor, P. (1980) 'The history of the present – contradiction and struggle in nursing', in *Rewriting Nursing History*, ed. C. Davies, Croom Helm, Beckenham.

Bendix, R. (1971) 'Bureaucracy' in *Scholarship and Partnership: Essays on Max Weber*. ed. R. Bendix and G. Roth, University of California Press, Berkeley.

Bendix, R. (1977) *Max Weber: An Intellectual Portrait*, Cambridge University Press, Cambridge.

Benjamin, M. & Curtis, J. (1981) *Ethics in Nursing*, Oxford University Press, Oxford.

Best, G. (1985) 'Keeping the district family happy.' *HSSJ*, **XCV** (4966).

Best, G. (1987) *The Future of NHS General Management: Where next?* King's Fund, London.

Billis, D. (1984) Welfare Bureaucracies, Heinemann, London.

Billis, D. & Rowbottom, R. (1987) *Organisational Design; the Work-Levels Approach*, Gower Press, Aldershot.

Blau, P. M. (1972) *The Dynamics of Bureaucracy*, Phoenix Press, Chicago.

Blau, P. M. & Scott, W. R. (1963) *Formal Organisations*, Routledge, London.

Bradbeer Report (1954) *Report of the Committee on the Internal Administration of Hospitals*, Ministry of Health, HMSO, London.

Briggs Report (1972) *Report of the Committee on Nursing*, Cmnd. 5115, HMSO, London.

Brim, O. G., Freeman, H. E., Levine, S. and Scotch, N. A. (1970) *The Dying Patient*, Russell Sage Foundation, New York.

Burns, T. & Stalker, G. M. (1961) *The Management of Innovation*, Tavistock Publications, London.

Calabresi, G. & Bobbitt, P. (1978) *Tragic Choices*, Norton & Co., New York.

Carpenter, M. (1977) 'The new managerialism and professionalism in nursing', in *Health and the Division of Labour*, ed. M. Stacey, M. Reid, C. Heath & R. Dingwall, Croom Helm, London.

Carpenter, M. (1978) 'Managerialism and the division of labour in nursing', in *Readings in the Sociology of Nursing*, ed. R. Dingwall & J. MacIntosh, Churchill Livingstone, London.

Carpenter, M. (1982) 'The Labour Movement in the National Health Service', in *Industrial Relations and Health Services*, ed. A. S. Sethi & S. J. Dimmock, Croom Helm, London.

Carrier, J. & Kendall, I. (1986) 'NHS Management and the Griffiths Report', in *Year Book of Social Policy 1985–6*, M. Brenton & C. Ungerson, Routledge, London.

Carr-Saunders, A. M. & Wilson, P. M. (1933) *The Professions*, Clarendon Press, Oxford.

Chiplin B. & Sloane P. J. (1982) *Tackling Discrimination in the Workplace: An Analysis of Sex Discrimination in Britain*, Cambridge University Press, Cambridge.

Cmnd. 247 (1987) *Promoting Better Health*, HMSO, London.

Cole, C. (1987) *Nursing in a Post-Griffiths World*, King's Fund College, London.

Committee of Public Accounts (1987) *Control of NHS Manpower*, HMSO, London.

Comptroller & Auditor General (1985) *The National Health Service: Control of Nursing Manpower*, HMSO, London.

Cookson, S. (1986) 'The politics of health: when the quality of mercy is strained', *Listener*, **116** (2972).

Crompton, S. (1988) 'Manchester consultants launch campaign for NHS', *HSJ*, **98** (5098).

Craig, J. (1983) 'The Growth of the Elderly Population', *Population Trends*, **32**.

Crossman, R. H. (1976) *Diaries of a Cabinet Minister*, Vol. 2. Hamilton and Cape, London.

Cumberlege Report (1986) *Neighbourhood Nursing – a Focus for Care*, Report of the Community Nursing Review, HMSO, London.

Davies, C. (1983) 'Professionals in bureaucracies: the conflict theory revisited', in *The Sociology of the Professions*, ed. R. Dingwall & P. Lewis, Macmillan, London.

Davies, C. & Rosser, J. (1986) *Processes of Discrimination: A Study of Women Working in the NHS*, DHSS, London.

Davis, F. (1968) 'Professional socialization as subjective experience', in *Institutions and the Person*, ed. H. A. Becker *et al.*, Aldine, Chicago.

Day, P. & Klein, R. (1983) 'Two Views of the Griffiths Report', *Brit. Med. J.*, **287** (6407) 1813–16.

Day, P. & Klein, R. (1986) 'That's the way the money goes' in *HSJ*, **96** (5027).

Delamothe, T. (1988) 'Nursing Grievances' *Brit. Med. J.*, **296,** pp. 25–8, 120–3, 182–5, 271–4, 345–7, 406–8.

DHSS (1970) *The Future of the National Health Service*, HMSO, London.

DHSS (1972) *Management Arrangements for the Reorganised National Health Service*, HMSO, London.

DHSS (1976) *Priorities for Health and Personal Social Services*, HMSO, London.

DHSS (1977) *Priorities for Health and Personal Social Services: A Way Forward*, HMSO, London.

DHSS (1984a) Implementing the NHS Inquiry Report. Questions and Answer Brief, HMSO, London.

DHSS (1984b) The Next Steps: Management in the Health Service, HMSO, London.

DHSS (1984c) *Implementing the NHS Inquiry Report*, Circular HC (84) 13.

Dingwall, R. & Lewis, P. (1983) *The Sociology of the Professions*, Macmillan, London.

Dingwall, R. & McIntosh, J. (1978) *Readings in the Sociology of Nursing*, Churchill Livingstone, London.

Disken, S., Dixon, M. & Halper, S. (1987) 'The new UGMs – an analysis of management at unit level' *HSJ*, **97** (5055).

Dixon, M. (1985) *Maximising Management Investment in the Health Service*, King's Fund College, London.

Douglas, M. (1987) *How Institutions Think*, Routledge & Kegan Paul, London.

Drucker, P. (1979) *Management*, Pan Books, London.

Dunea, G. (1988) 'Nurse's shortages.' *Brit. Med. J.*, **296**, 911–12.

Dunleavy, P. (1987) *Theories of the State*, Macmillan, London.

Dunn, A. (1986) 'Nursing a real grievance over management', *HSJ*, **96** (4983).

Eckstein, H. (1958) *The English Health Service*, Harvard University Press, Cambridge, Mass.

Elliot, B. (1988) 'Repeating the same old story', *HSJ*, **98** (5085).

Enthoven, A. C. (1985) *Reflections on the Management of the NHS*, Nuffield, Occasional Paper No. 5, Provincial Hospitals Trust, Oxford.

Etzioni, A. (1969) *The Semi Professions and their Organisations*, Free Press, New York.

Evans, T. (1983) *Griffiths – the Right Prescription?*, CIPFA, London.

Farquharson-Lang Report (1966) *Administrative Practice of Hospital Boards in Scotland*. Scottish Home and Health Department, HMSO, London.

Fayol, H. (1949) *General Industrial Management*, Pitman, London.

Feinmann, J. (1988) 'Four hospitals into one might go', *HSJ*, **98** (5087).

Friedman, M. (1962) *Capitalism and Freedom*, University of Chicago Press.

Game, A. & Pringle, R. (1983) *Gender at Work*, Pluto Press, London.

Gapper, J. (1988) 'Nurses in RCN warned against joining strikes', *Financial Times*, 22 January.

Garmarnikow, E. (1978) 'The Sexual Division of Labour: the Case of Nursing', in *Feminism and Materialism*, ed. A. Kuhn & A. M. Wolpe, Routledge & Kegan Paul, London.

Glaser B. G. & Strauss, A. L. (1979) 'Dying on time', in *Where Medicine Fails*, ed. A. L. Strauss, Transaction Books, New Jersey.

Glennerster, H. (1974) *Social Service Budgets and Social Policy*, Allen & Unwin, London.

Glennerster, H. (1983) *Planning for Priority Groups*. Martin Robertson, Oxford.

Glennerster, H. & Owens, P. (1986) *The Nursing Management Function after Griffiths*, NWT & LSE, London.

Glennerster, H. & Owens, P. (1987) *The Nursing Management Function after Griffiths: Second Interim Report*, NWT & LSE, London.

Gluckmann, M. (1970) *Custom and Conflict in Africa*, Blackwell, Oxford.

Goldsmith, M. & Willetts, D. (1988) *Managed Health Care: A New System for Better Health Service*,

Gorer, G. (1965) *Death Grief and Mourning in Contemporary Britain*, The Cresset Press, London.

Griffiths Report (1983) *Recommendations on the Effective use of Manpower and Related Resources*, HMSO, London.

Guillebaud Report (1956) *Report of the Committee of Inquiry into the Cost of the National Health Service*, Cmnd. 9663, HMSO, London.

Hall, R. H. (1977) *Organisations: Structure and Process*, Prentice Hall, New Jersey.

Ham, C. (1985) *Health Policy in Britain*, Macmillan, London, pp. 45, 65–8.

Hildrew, P. (1987a) 'The nursing scandal', *Guardian*, November.

Hildrew, P. (1987b) 'Nurses offered raw deal', *Guardian*, 19 December.

Hill, G. (1988) 'A lamp still burning', *The Times*, 2 February.

Hillingdon Health Authority (1987) *Review of Nursing Services Report*.

House of Commons (1984) *First Report from the Social Services Committee – Griffiths NHS Management Inquiry Report March 1984*, H.C. 209, HMSO, London.

House of Commons (1986) *Report of the Social Services Committee*, HMSO, London.

House of Commons (1987) *Public Expenditure on the Social Services*, Social Services Committee, session 1986–7, HMSO, London.

Hoyland, P. (1987) 'Too efficient doctors must treat fewer cases', *Guardian*, 27 November.

Hughes, E. (1958) *Men and their Work*, The Free Press, Glencoe.

Hunter, M. (1988) 'Coping with uncertainty: policy and politics in the NHS', *Social Policy Research Monograph 2*, Research Studies Press, Hertfordshire.

Illich, I. (1977) *Medical Nemesis*, Penguin, Harmondsworth.

Independent (1988) 'Trevor Clay, embattled leader of the RCN', Weekend Profile, 6 February.

Jacques, E. (1978) *Health Services: Their Nature and Organisation*, Heinemann, London.

Jones, M. (1988) 'Health: cabinet turns on Moore', *The Times*, 17 January.

Kellehear, A. (1984) 'Are we a death-denying society? A Sociological Review', *Soc. Sci. Med.*, **18 (9),** 713–23.

Kenny, D. (1988) Kings Fund Seminar, June 1988.

King's Fund (1987) *London's Health Services*, King's Fund, London.

King's Fund Institute (1988) *Health Finance; Assessing the Options*, King's Fund Institute, London.

Kinston, W. (1987) *Stronger Nursing Organisation*, Brunel University, Alton.

Klein, R. (1983) *The Politics of the National Health Service*, Longman, London.

Lees, D. (1967) *The Economic Consequences of the Professions*, Institute of Economic Affairs, London.

Leininger, M. M. (1970) *Nursing and Anthropology: Two Worlds Blend*, Wiley & Sons, Chichester.

Letwin, O. & Redwood, J. (1988) *Britain's Biggest Enterprise: Ideas for Radical Reform of the NHS*, Centre for Policy Studies, London.

Lévi-Strauss, C. (1977) *Structural Anthropology*, Penguin, Harmondsworth.

Levine, C. H. (1978) 'Organisational decline and cutback management', *Public Administration Review*, July/August.

Levine S. & Scotch N. A. (1970) 'Dying as an emerging social problem', in *The Dying Patient*, ed. O. G. Brimm *et al.*, Russell Sage Foundation, New York.

Lewis, J. (1987) *What Price Community Medicine?* Wheatsheaf, Brighton.

Machiavelli, N. (1513) *The Prince*. English translation (1979) in *The Portable Machiavelli*, ed. P. Bondanella & M. Musa, Penguin, Harmondsworth.

Malinowski, B. (1974) *Magic, Science & Religion and other essays*, Souvenir Press, London.

Maynard, A. (1984) 'Perspectives in NHS management'. *Brit. Med. J.*, **288** (6422).

Maynard, A. (1987a) 'Is the NHS underfinanced?', *HSJ*, **97** (5067).

Maynard, A. (1987b) 'Logic in Medicine: an economic perspective', *Brit. Med. J.*, **295** (6612).

Maynard, A. (1987c) What nursing shortage? *HSJ*, **97** (5071).

Maynard, A. (1987d) 'Who cares about the NHS?', *HSJ*, **97** (5079).

Mays, N. & Bevan, G. (1987) *Resource Allocation in the National Health Service*. Occasional Papers in Social Administration *Health*, No. 81, Bedford Square Press, London.

Mayston Report (1969) *Report of the UK Working Party on the Management Structure of Local Authority Nursing Services*, HMSO, London.

Melia, K. (1987) *Learning and Working: The Occupational Socialisation of Nurses*, Tavistock Publications, London.

Melosh, B. (1986) 'Nursing and Reagonomics: Lost Containment in the United States', in *Political Issues in Nursing: Past, Present and Future*, Vol. 2, ed. R. White, Wiley, Chichester.

Mercer, G. M. (1979) *The Employment of Nurses*, Croom Helm, Beckenham.

Merifield, A. S. (1987) *Letter to Regional General Managers, 27.2.87*, DHSS, London.

Millar, B. (1988) 'Health Service cuts: the right to speak out', *HSJ*, **98** (5109).

Moores, B. (1987) 'The changing composition of the British hospital nursing workforce 1962–84', *J. Adv. Nursing*, 499–504.

Mueller, C. W. (1981) *Professional Turnover: the Case of Nurses*, Health Systems Management, vol. 15, Spectrum, New York.

Mueller, D. (1979) *Public Choice*, Cambridge University Press, Cambridge.

Muff, J. (1982) 'Handmaiden, battle-axe or whore: An exploration into fantasies, myths and stereotypes about nurses', in *Socialisation, Sexism, and Stereotyping: Womens Issues in Nursing*, ed. J. Muff, Mosby, St. Louis.

Murray, A. (1986) *An Analysis of the General Management Function Prescribed for the NHS*, Sheffield City Polytechnic.

NAHA (1983) Conference Report, *Hospital & Social Services News*, 17 August.

NHS *Management Bulletin* (1987) 'Fairer Deal for Women Employees', Issue No. 8.

Nicholson-Lord, D. (1988) 'Young set on high-earning careers', *The Times*, 2 September.

Nightingale, F. (1859) *Notes on Nursing: What it is, and what it is not*. Reprinted (1980), Churchill Livingstone, Edinburgh.

NIHSM, BMA & RCN (1983) *Public Expenditure in the NHS: Recent Trends and Outlook*. Joint Report, London.

NUPE & LPU (1987) *Nursing and Grievance: Low Pay in Nursing*, National Union of Public Employees/Low Pay Unit, London.

Nursing Mirror (1983) Editorial, 'New-Look NHS threatens voice', **157** (18), 2 November.

Nursing Mirror (1984) News, 'Nursing bodies unite to condemn business-style management plan', **158** (3), 18 January.

Nursing Times (1985) News, **81** (25), 19 June.

Nursing Times (1987) Interview with Sir Roy Griffiths, **83** (31), 12 August.

Nursing Times (1988a) 'Map of nursing establishments and shortages', **84** (4).

Nursing Times (1988b) News, 'Regrading may cost extra £150m.', **84** (34).

Nuttall, P. (1987) 'Male Takeover or Female Giveaway', *Nursing Times*, **79** (2).

Nutting, M.A. & Dock, L.L. (1907) *A History of Nursing*, G.P. Putnam's Sons, London.

NWTRHA (1987) *Towards a Strategy for Dying and Bereaved People*, Regional Strategy, NWTHA, London.

Oakley, R. (1988) 'Bitter row as Thatcher hits at NHS strike', *The Times*, 22 February.

OECD (1985) *Measuring Health Care 1960–83*, OECD, Paris.

OECD (1987) *Financing and Delivering Health Care*, OECD, Paris.

Peet, J. (1987) *Healthy Competition: How to Improve the NHS*, Centre for Policy Studies, London.

Pembrey, S. (1980) *The Ward Sister: Key to Nursing*, RCN, London.

Peters, T.S., & Waterman, R.H. (1982) *In Search of Excellence: Lessons from America's Best-Run Companies*, Harper & Row, New York.

Pickering, M. and Fox, P. (1987) 'The ward manager', *Health Care Management*, **2** (3), 23–26.

Pirie, M. & Butler, E. (1988) *The Health of Nations*, Adam Smith Institute, London.

Plant, J. 'Sole Charge of the Ward', *HSSJ*, **XCV** (4967), 1198.

Pondy, L.R. (1983) 'Psyche and symbolism', in *Organisational Symbolism*, ed. L.R. Pondy, JAI Press, Greenwich, Connecticut.

Prentice, W. (1988) Letter to *The Times*, 14 October.

Price, M. & Butler, E. (1988) *The Health of Nations*, Adam Smith Institute, London.

Price-Waterhouse (1988) *Nurse Retention and Recruitment: A Matter of Priority*, Price-Waterhouse, London.

RCN Advertisement (1986) *The Times*, 12 January.

RCN Advertisement (1986) *The Times*, 14 January.

RCN Advertisement (1986) *Guardian*, 21 January.

Reuschemeyer, D. (1983) Professional autonomy & the social control of expertise, in *The Sociology of the Professions*, eds. R. Dingwall and P. Lewis, Macmillan, London.

Review Body for Nursing Staff, Midwives, Health Visitors and Allied Professions to Medicine, 5th Report (1988) Cmnd. 360, HMSO, London.

Robinson, J. & Strong, P. (1988) *New Model Management: Griffiths and the NHS*, Nursing Studies Policy Centre, Warwick University.

Rosenthal, C.J. (1980) *Nurses, Patients and Families*, Croom Helm, London.

Royal Commission on the NHS (1979), Report, Cmnd. 7615, HMSO, London.

Salmon Report (1966) *Report of the Committee on Senior Nursing Staff Structure*, Ministry of Health, HMSO, London.

Salvage, J. (1985) *The Politics of Nursing*, Heinemann, London.

Schurr, M.C. & Turner, J. (1982) *Nursing – Image or Reality*, Hodder & Stoughton, Sevenoaks.

Scott, W. R. (1964) 'Theory of Organisations', in *Handbook of Modern Sociology*, ed. R. E. L. Farris, Rand McNally, Chicago.

Scott, W. R. & Meyer, J. W. (1983) *Organisational Environments: Ritual and Rationality*, Sage, London.

Seton, C. (1987a) 'Heart boy too ill for hospital switch', *The Times*, 24 November.

Seton, C. (1987b) 'Baby dies awaiting treatment', *The Times*, 25 November.

Sherman, J. (1987) 'NHS losing specialists to private hospitals', *The Times*, 15 October.

Sherman, J. (1988a) 'Government's aim is a free nurses' market', *The Times*, 7 February.

Sherman, J. (1988b) 'Nine nurses trained to fill 500 vital intensive care jobs', *The Times*, 22 February.

Sherman, J. (1988c) 'Experience and skill bring extra reward for nurses', *The Times*, 22 April.

Sherman, J. (1988d) 'Government move to defuse nursing pay crisis', *The Times*, 12 August.

Sherman, J. (1988e) 'Nurses protest at annual pay policy', *The Times*, 5 October.

Stacey, M., Reid, M., Heath, C. & Dingwall, R. (1977) *Health and the Division of Labour*, Croom Helm, London.

Stewart, R. & Shermon, J. (1967) *Continuously Under Review*, Occasional Paper in Social Administration, No. 20., Bell, London.

Strauss, A. L. (1979) *Where Medicine Fails*, Transaction Books, New Jersey.

Strauss, A. L. (1969) *Mirrors and Masks: The Search for Identity*, The Sociology Press, California.

Templeton College (1987) *Managing Better Health: Series on District General Managers*, Oxford Centre for Management Studies.

The Times (1987) Law Report, 26 November.

Timmins, N. & Spackman, A. (1987) 'Rising toll of bed closures', *Independent*, 9 December.

Tongue, C. (1986) 'Why a lot of Directors are imposters', *Guardian*, 21 August.

UKCC (1986) *Project 2000: A New Preparation for Practice*, UK Central Council for Nursing Midwifery and Health Visiting, London.

Van Gennep, A. (1960) *The Rites of Passage*, Routledge & Kegan Paul, London.

Veitch, A. (1987a) 'A grief of nurses', *Guardian*, 26 November.

Veitch, A. (1987b) 'Two more children die after hospital delays in heart operations', *Guardian*, 6 December.

Walter, G. A. (1983) 'Psyche & Symbol', in *Organisational Symbolism*, ed. L. R. Pondy *et al.*, JAI Press, London.

Weber, M. (1947) *The Theory of Social and Economic Organisation*, Free Press, New York.

Webster, C. (1988) *The Health Services Since the War*, HMSO, London.

Webster, P. (1988) MP suspended after health cut uproar', *The Times*, 12 January.

White, R. (1986) *Political Issues in Nursing Vol. 2*, John Wiley & Sons Ltd., Chichester.

White, R. (1984) 'Altruism is not enough: barriers in the development of nursing as a profession', *J. Adv. Nursing*, **9** (6) 555–62.

Whittaker E. & Olsen V. (1978) 'The faces of Florence Nightingale: the functions of the heroine legend in the occupational subculture', in *Readings in the Sociology of Nursing*, ed. R. Dingwall & J. MacIntosh, Churchill Livingstone, London.

Wilding, P. (1982) *Professional Power and Social Welfare*, Routledge & Kegan Paul, London.

Willetts, D. & Goldsmith, M. (1988) *A Mixed-Economy in Health Care; more spending less taxes*, Centre for Policy Studies, London.

Williamson, J. (1986) 'Keeping the trainees taped', *HSSJ*, **96** (4987).

Wood, N. & Sherman, J. (1988) 'More funds for nurses' pay', *The Times*, 14 October.

Woodham-Smith, C. (1951) *Florence Nightingale 1820–1910*, Collins, London.

Young, A. P. (1981) *Legal Problems in Nursing Practice*, Harper & Row, London.

Index

———————— ◆ ————————

176